CONTENTS

CLASSIC DAILY BREAD

Oat Quinoa Bread

Servings: 1 Loaf
Ingredients:

- 16 slice bread (2 pounds)
- 1⅓ cups lukewarm milk
- ¾ cup cooked quinoa, cooled
- 5 tablespoons unsalted butter, melted
- 4 teaspoons sugar
- 1⅓ teaspoons table salt
- 2 cups white bread flour
- 5 tablespoons quick oats
- 1 cup whole-wheat flour
- 2 teaspoons bread machine yeast
- 12 slice bread (1½ pounds)
- 1 cup lukewarm milk
- ⅔ cup cooked quinoa, cooled
- ¼ cup unsalted butter, melted
- 1 tablespoon sugar
- 1 teaspoon table salt
- 1½ cups white bread flour
- ¼ cup quick oats
- ¾ cup whole-wheat flour
- 1½ teaspoons bread machine yeast

Directions:

1. Choose the size of loaf you would like to make and measure your ingredients.
2. Add the ingredients to the bread pan in the order listed above.
3. Place the pan in the bread machine and close the lid.
4. Turn on the bread maker. Select the White/Basic setting, then the loaf size, and finally the crust color. Start the cycle.
5. When the cycle is finished and the bread is baked, carefully remove the pan from the machine. Use a potholder as the handle will be very hot. Let rest for a few minutes.
6. Remove the bread from the pan and allow to cool on a wire rack for at least 10 minutes before slicing.

Nutrition Info: (Per Serving):Calories 153, fat 5.3 g, carbs 22.3 g, sodium 238 mg, protein 3.8 g

Chocolate Chip Bread

Servings: 14 Slices
Cooking Time: 3 H.
Ingredients:

- ¼ cup water
- 1 cup milk
- 1 egg
- 3 cups bread flour
- 3 Tbsp brown sugar
- 2 Tbsp white sugar
- 1 tsp salt
- 1 tsp ground cinnamon
- 1½ tsp active dry yeast
- 2 Tbsp margarine, softened
- ¾ cup semisweet chocolate chips

Directions:

1. Add each ingredient except the chocolate chips to the bread machine in the order and at the temperature recommended by your bread machine manufacturer.
2. Close the lid, select the sweet loaf, low crust setting on your bread machine, and press start.
3. Add the chocolate chips about 5 minutes before the kneading cycle has finished.
4. When the bread machine has finished baking, remove the bread and put it on a cooling rack.

Rosemary Focaccia Bread

Servings: 4 - 6
Cooking Time: 3 Hours
Ingredients:

- 1 cup, plus 3 tablespoons water
- 1 tablespoon extra-virgin olive oil
- 1 teaspoon salt
- 2 teaspoons fresh rosemary, chopped
- 3 cups bread flour
- 1 1/2 teaspoons instant yeast
- For the topping:
- 3 tablespoons olive oil
- Coarse salt
- Red pepper flakes

Directions:

1. Add water, oil, salt, rosemary, and flour to the bread maker pan.
2. Make a well in the center of the dry ingredients and add the yeast.
3. Select Dough cycle and press Start.
4. Transfer finished dough to a floured surface.
5. Cover and let rest for 5 minutes.
6. Form dough into a smooth ball and roll into a 12-inch round.
7. Place on a 12-inch pizza pan that has been lightly greased with olive oil. Poke dough randomly with fingertips to form dimples. Brush top with olive oil and sprinkle with salt and red pepper flakes to taste.
8. Let rise uncovered in warm, draft-free space for about 30 minutes.
9. Bake at 425°F for 18 to 22 minutes or until done.
10. Serve warm.

Nutrition Info: Calories: 312, Sodium: 390 mg, Dietary Fiber: 2.1 g, Fat: 10.1 g, Carbs: 48.3 g, Protein: 6.9 g.

Onion Bread

Servings: 12
Cooking Time: 3 Hours And 25 Minutes
Ingredients:
- Water – 1 ½ cup
- Butter – 2 tbsp. plus 2 tsp.
- Salt – 1 tsp.
- Sugar – 1 tbsp. plus 1 ½ tsp.
- Bread flour – 4 cups
- Nonfat dry milk – 2 tbsp. plus 2 tsp.
- Active dry yeast – 2 tsp.
- Dry onion soup mix – 4 tbsp.

Directions:
1. Place ingredients in the bread pan in the order listed, except the soup.
2. Select Basic cycle. Add the onion soup mix at the fruit and nut signal.
3. When done, remove and cool.
4. Slice and serve.

Nutrition Info: (Per Serving): Calories: 130; Total Fat: 3 g; Saturated Fat: 2 g; Carbohydrates: 16 g; Cholesterol: 8 mg; Fiber: 1 g; Calcium: 77 mg; Sodium: 843 mg; Protein: 8 g

Tomato Basil Bread

Servings: 16
Cooking Time: 4 Hours
Ingredients:
- 3/4 cup warm water
- 1/4 cup fresh basil, minced
- 1/4 cup parmesan cheese, grated
- 3 tablespoons tomato paste
- 1 tablespoon sugar
- 1 tablespoon olive oil
- 1 teaspoon salt
- 1/4 teaspoon crushed red pepper flakes
- 2 1/2 cups bread flour
- 1 package active dry yeast
- Flour, for surface

Directions:
1. Add ingredients, except yeast, to bread maker pan in above listed order.
2. Make a well in the flour; pour the yeast into the hole.
3. Select Dough cycle and press Start.
4. Turn finished dough out onto a floured surface and knead until smooth and elastic, about 3 to 5 minutes.
5. Place in a greased bowl, turning once to grease top. Cover and let rise in a warm place until doubled, about 1 hour.
6. Punch dough down and knead for 1 minute.
7. Shape into a round loaf. Place on a greased baking sheet. Cover and let rise until doubled, about 1 hour.
8. With a sharp knife, cut a large "X" in top of loaf. Bake at 375°F for 35-40 minutes or until golden brown.
9. Remove from pan and cool on a cooling rack before serving.

Nutrition Info: Calories: 91, Sodium: 172 mg, Dietary Fiber: 0.8 g, Fat: 1.5 g, Carbs: 16.5 g, Protein: 2.8 g.

Oat Bran Nutmeg Bread

Servings: 1 Loaf
Ingredients:
- 16 slice bread (2 pounds)
- 1 cup lukewarm water

- 3 tablespoons unsalted butter, melted
- ¼ cup blackstrap molasses
- ½ teaspoon table salt
- 3 cups whole-wheat bread flour
- ¼ teaspoon ground nutmeg
- 1 cup oat bran
- 2¼ teaspoons bread machine yeast
- 12 slice bread (1½ pounds)
- ¾ cup lukewarm water
- 2¼ tablespoons unsalted butter, melted
- 3 tablespoons blackstrap molasses
- ⅓ teaspoon table salt
- 2¼ cups whole-wheat bread flour
- ¼ teaspoon ground nutmeg
- ¾ cup oat bran
- 1⅔ teaspoons bread machine yeast

Directions:

1. Choose the size of loaf you would like to make and measure your ingredients.
2. Add the ingredients to the bread pan in the order listed above.
3. Place the pan in the bread machine and close the lid.
4. Turn on the bread maker. Select the Whole Wheat/Wholegrain setting, then the loaf size, and finally the crust color. Start the cycle.
5. When the cycle is finished and the bread is baked, carefully remove the pan from the machine. Use a potholder as the handle will be very hot. Let rest for a few minutes.
6. Remove the bread from the pan and allow to cool on a wire rack for at least 10 minutes before slicing.

Nutrition Info: (Per Serving):Calories 141, fat 2.8 g, carbs 23.6 g, sodium 124 mg, protein 3.4 g

Sausage Herb And Onion Bread

Servings: 14 Slices
Cooking Time: 3 H. 10 Min.

Ingredients:

- ¾ tsp basil leaves
- 1½ Tbsp sugar
- ⅜ cup wheat bran
- 1 medium onion, minced
- 2¼ tsp yeast
- ¾ tsp rosemary leaves
- ½ Tbsp salt
- 1½ Tbsp parmesan, grated
- 3 cups bread flour
- ¾ tsp oregano leaves
- ¾ tsp thyme leaves
- 1⅛ cups water
- ¾ cup Italian sausage

Directions:

1. Remove casing from sausage. Crumble the meat into a medium nonstick skillet.
2. Cook on medium heat, stirring and breaking up sausage until it begins to render its juices.
3. Add onion and cook for 2-3 minuts until it softens and the sausage is no longer pink.
4. Remove from heat and let it cool.
5. Add each ingredient to the bread machine in the order and at the temperature recommended by your bread machine manufacturer.
6. Close the lid, select the basic bread, medium crust setting on your bread machine, and press start.
7. When the bread machine has finished baking, remove the bread and put it on a cooling rack.

Whole Wheat Sunflower Bread

Servings: 1 Loaf

Ingredients:

- 16 slice bread (2 pounds)
- 1⅛ cups lukewarm water
- 2 tablespoons honey
- 2 tablespoons unsalted butter, melted
- 1 teaspoon table salt
- 3 cups whole-wheat flour
- 1 cup white bread flour
- 2 tablespoons sesame seeds
- ¼ cup raw sunflower seeds
- 2¼ teaspoons bread machine yeast
- 12 slice bread (1½ pounds)
- 1 cup lukewarm water
- 1½ tablespoons honey
- 1½ tablespoons unsalted butter, melted
- ¾ teaspoon table salt
- 2½ cups whole-wheat flour
- ¾ cup white bread flour
- 1 tablespoon sesame seeds

- 3 tablespoons raw sunflower seeds
- 1½ teaspoons bread machine yeast

Directions:

1. Choose the size of loaf you would like to make and measure your ingredients.
2. Add the ingredients to the bread pan in the order listed above.
3. Place the pan in the bread machine and close the lid.
4. Turn on the bread maker. Select the Whole Wheat/Wholegrain setting, then the loaf size, and finally the crust color. Start the cycle.
5. When the cycle is finished and the bread is baked, carefully remove the pan from the machine. Use a potholder as the handle will be very hot. Let rest for a few minutes.
6. Remove the bread from the pan and allow to cool on a wire rack for at least 10 minutes before slicing.

Nutrition Info: (Per Serving):Calories 253, fat 3.3 g, carbs 27.4 g, sodium 154 mg, protein 4.2 g

Insane Coffee Cake

Servings: 10 - 12
Cooking Time: 2 Hours
Ingredients:

- 7/8 cup of milk
- 1/4 cup of sugar
- 1 teaspoon salt
- 1 egg yolk
- 1 tablespoon butter
- 2 1/4 cups bread flour
- 2 teaspoons of active dry yeast
- For the topping:
- 2 tablespoons butter, melted
- 2 tablespoons brown sugar
- 1 teaspoon cinnamon

Directions:

1. Set the topping ingredients aside and add the rest of the ingredients to the bread pan in the order above.
2. Set the bread machine to the Dough cycle.
3. Butter a 9-by-9-inch glass baking dish and pour the dough into the dish. Cover with a towel and let rise for about 10 minutes.
4. Preheat an oven to 375°F.

5. Brush the dough with the melted butter.
6. Mix the brown sugar and cinnamon in a bowl and sprinkle on top of the coffee cake.
7. Let the topped dough rise, uncovered, for another 30 minutes.
8. Place in oven and bake for 30 to 35 minutes or until a wooden toothpick inserted into the center comes out clean and dry.
9. When baked, let the coffee cake rest for 10 minutes. Carefully remove the coffee cake from the dish with a rubber spatula, slice and serve.

Nutrition Info: Calories: 148, Sodium: 211 mg, Dietary Fiber: 0.9 g, Fat: 3.9 g, Carbs: 24.9 g, Protein: 3.5 g.

Buttermilk Bread

Servings: 1 Loaf
Ingredients:

- 16 slice bread (2 pounds)
- 1¼ cups lukewarm buttermilk
- 2 tablespoons unsalted butter, melted
- 2 tablespoons sugar
- 1½ teaspoons table salt
- ½ teaspoon baking powder
- 3½ cups white bread flour
- 2¼ teaspoons bread machine yeast
- 12 slice bread (1½ pounds)
- 1¼ cups lukewarm buttermilk
- 1½ tablespoons unsalted butter, melted
- 1½ tablespoons sugar
- 1⅛ teaspoons table salt
- ⅓ teaspoon baking powder
- 2⅔ cups white bread flour
- 1⅔ teaspoons bread machine yeast

Directions:

1. Choose the size of loaf you would like to make and measure your ingredients.
2. Add the ingredients to the bread pan in the order listed above.
3. Place the pan in the bread machine and close the lid.
4. Turn on the bread maker. Select the White/Basic setting, then the loaf size, and finally the crust color. Start the cycle.
5. When the cycle is finished and the bread is baked, carefully remove the pan from the machine.

Use a potholder as the handle will be very hot. Let rest for a few minutes.

6. Remove the bread from the pan and allow to cool on a wire rack for at least 10 minutes before slicing.

Nutrition Info: (Per Serving):Calories 132, fat 2.2 g, carbs 23.4 g, sodium 234 mg, protein 4.3 g

Carrot Cake Bread

Servings: 12 - 16
Cooking Time: 1 Hours 20 Minutes
Ingredients:
- Non-stick cooking spray
- 1/4 cup vegetable oil
- 2 large eggs, room temperature
- 1/2 teaspoon pure vanilla extract
- 1/2 cup sugar
- 1/4 cup light brown sugar
- 1/4 cup crushed pineapple with juice (from can or fresh)
- 1 1/4 cups unbleached, all-purpose flour
- 1 teaspoon baking powder
- 1/4 teaspoon baking soda
- 1/4 teaspoon salt
- 1 teaspoon ground cloves
- 3/4 teaspoon ground cinnamon
- 1 cup freshly grated carrots
- 1/3 cup chopped pecans
- 1/3 cup golden raisins

Directions:
1. Coat the inside of the bread pan with non-stick cooking spray.
2. Add all of the ingredients, in order listed, to the bread pan.
3. Select Express Bake, medium crust color, and press Start. While the batter is mixing, scrape the sides of the bread pan with a rubber spatula to fully incorporate ingredients.
4. When baked, remove from bread pan and place on wire rack to cool completely before slicing and serving.

Nutrition Info: Calories: 151, Sodium: 69 mg, Dietary Fiber: 1.2 g, Fat: 7.2 g, Carbs: 20.1 g, Protein: 2.4 g.

Coffee Rye Bread

Servings: 6
Cooking Time: 3 Hours And 25 Minutes
Ingredients:
- Lukewarm water – ½ cup
- Brewed coffee – ¼ cup, 80ºF
- Dark molasses – 2 tbsp.
- Brown sugar – 5 tsp.
- Unsalted butter – 4 tsp., softened
- Powdered skim milk – 1 tbsp.
- Kosher salt – 1 tsp.
- Unsweetened cocoa powder – 4 tsp.
- Dark rye flour – 2/3 cup
- Whole-wheat bread machine flour – ½ cup
- Caraway seeds – 1 tsp.
- White bread machine flour – 1 cup
- Bread machine yeast – 1 ½ tsp

Directions:
1. Place everything in the bread machine pan according to the bread machine recommendation.
2. Select Basic and Light crust. Press Start.
3. Remove the bread.
4. Cool, slice, and serve.

Nutrition Info: (Per Serving): Calories: 222; Total Fat: 3.2 g; Saturated Fat: 1.8 g; Carbohydrates: 42.9 g; Cholesterol: 8 mg; Fiber: 4.7 g; Calcium: 40 mg; Sodium: 415 mg; Protein: 6.3 g

Fat-free Whole Wheat Bread

Servings: 12
Cooking Time: 1 Hour And 20 Minutes
Ingredients:
- Water – 1 7/8 cup
- White whole wheat flour – 4 2/3 cups
- Vital wheat gluten – 4 tbsp.
- Sugar – 2 tbsp.
- Salt – 1 ½ tsp.
- Rapid rise yeast – 2 ½ tsp.

Directions:
1. Add the water in the bread machine pan.
2. Add the remaining ingredients according to bread machine recommendation.
3. Choose Quick-Bake Whole Wheat cycle and press Start.
4. Remove the bread when complete.

5. Cool, slice, and serve.

Nutrition Info: (Per Serving): Calories: 134; Total Fat: 0.6 g; Saturated Fat: 0 g; Carbohydrates: 27.6 g; Cholesterol: 11 mg; Fiber: 6.5 g; Calcium: 18 mg; Sodium: 221.5 mg; Protein: 6.5 g

Julekake

Servings: 14 Slices
Cooking Time: 3 H.
Ingredients:
- ⅓ cup evaporated milk
- ⅔ cup water
- 1 egg, room temperature
- 3⅓ cups bread flour
- ¼ cup sugar
- ½ tsp salt
- ½ tsp cardamom
- ½ cup softened butter, cut up
- 2¼ tsp dry active yeast
- ½ cup golden raisins
- ⅔ cup candied fruit

Directions:
1. Add each ingredient except the raisins to the bread machine in the order and at the temperature recommended by your bread machine manufacturer.
2. Close the lid, select the basic bread, low crust setting on your bread machine, and press start.
3. Add the raisins and fruit about 5 minutes before the kneading cycle has finished.
4. When the bread machine has finished baking, remove the bread and put it on a cooling rack.

Pumpernickel Bread

Servings: 1 Loaf
Ingredients:
- 16 slice bread (2 pounds)
- 1 1/3 cups water, lukewarm between 80 and 90⁰F
- 2 large eggs, room temperature and not cold
- ¼ cup oil
- ¼ cup honey
- 3 tablespoons dry milk powder
- ¼ cup cocoa powder
- 3 tablespoons caraway seeds
- 1 tablespoon instant coffee granules

- 2 teaspoons table salt
- 1 cup rye flour
- 1 cup whole wheat bread flour
- 2 cups white bread flour
- 2 ¼ teaspoons bread machine yeast
- 12 slice bread (1 ½ pounds)
- 3/4 cups water, lukewarm between 80 and 90⁰F
- 2 large eggs, room temperature and not cold
- 2 tablespoons oil
- 2 tablespoons honey
- 3 tablespoons dry milk powder
- 3 tablespoons cocoa powder
- 2 tablespoons caraway seeds
- 2 teaspoon instant coffee granules
- 1 1/2 teaspoons table salt
- 3/4 cup rye flour
- 3/4 cup whole wheat bread flour
- 1 1/2 cups white bread flour
- 1 3/4 teaspoons bread machine yeast

Directions:
1. Choose the size of loaf you would like to make and measure your ingredients. If you want to make a 1-pound or 2 ½-pound loaf, please adjust your ingredient quantities accordingly. You can look at the conversion table at the end of the book for easy adjustments or click here.
2. Take the bread pan; add the ingredients in order listed above.
3. Secure the pan into the bread machine and close the lid.
4. Power the bread maker and select the option of the bread – White/Basic – then the size of the loaf you are making, and finally the crust color you desire. Start the machine.
5. After the bread cycle is done and the bread is cooked, carefully remove the pan from the machine. Use a potholder as the handle will be very hot. Let rest for a few minutes.
6. Remove the bread from the pan and allow to cool down on a wired rack for at least 10 minutes or more before slicing.

Nutrition Info: (Per Serving):Calories 134, fat 3.1 g, carbs 19 g, sodium 143 mg, protein 4.2 g

French Bread

Servings: 8
Cooking Time: 3 Hours And 35 Minutes
Ingredients:
- Water - ⅔ cup
- Olive oil - 2 tsp.
- Sugar - 1 tbsp.
- Salt - ⅔ tsp.
- White bread flour - 2 cups
- Bread machine or instant yeast - 1 tsp.

Directions:
1. Place everything in the bread machine according to machine recommendation.
2. Press French bread and Light or Medium crust. Press Start.
3. Remove the loaf from the machine and cool.
4. Slice and serve.

Nutrition Info: (Per Serving): Calories: 135; Total Fat: 2 g; Saturated Fat: 0 g; Carbohydrates: 26 g; Cholesterol: 13 mg; Fiber: 1 g; Calcium: 17 mg; Sodium: 245 mg; Protein: 3 g

Rye Bread

Servings: 1 Loaf
Ingredients:
- 16 slice bread (2 pounds)
- 1⅔ cups lukewarm water
- ¼ cup + 4 teaspoons Dijon mustard
- 2 tablespoons unsalted butter, melted
- 4 teaspoons sugar
- 1 teaspoon table salt
- 2 cups rye flour
- 2⅔ cups white bread flour
- 1½ teaspoons bread machine yeast
- 12 slice bread (1½ pounds)
- 1¼ cups lukewarm water
- ¼ cup Dijon mustard
- 1½ tablespoons unsalted butter, melted
- 1 tablespoon sugar
- ¾ teaspoon table salt
- 1½ cups rye flour
- 2 cups white bread flour
- 1 teaspoon bread machine yeast

Directions:

1. Choose the size of loaf you would like to make and measure your ingredients.
2. Add the ingredients to the bread pan in the order listed above.
3. Place the pan in the bread machine and close the lid.
4. Turn on the bread maker. Select the White/Basic setting, then the loaf size, and finally the crust color. Start the cycle.
5. When the cycle is finished and the bread is baked, carefully remove the pan from the machine. Use a potholder as the handle will be very hot. Let rest for a few minutes.
6. Remove the bread from the pan and allow to cool on a wire rack for at least 10 minutes before slicing.

Nutrition Info: (Per Serving):Calories 153, fat 2.1 g, carbs 24.8 g, sodium 256 mg, protein 5.2 g

Lemon Blueberry Quick Bread

Servings: 10 - 12
Cooking Time: 2 Hours
Ingredients:
- 2 cups all-purpose flour
- 1 1/2 teaspoons baking powder
- 1/2 teaspoon salt
- 1 tablespoon lemon zest
- 1 cup sugar
- 1/2 cup unsalted butter, softened
- 2 large eggs
- 2 teaspoons pure vanilla extract
- 1/2 cup whole milk
- 1 1/2 cups blueberries
- For the crumb topping:
- 1/3 cup sugar
- 3 tablespoons all-purpose flour
- 2 tablespoons butter, melted
- Non-stick cooking spray

Directions:
1. Spray bread maker pan with non-stick cooking spray and lightly flour.
2. Combine crumb topping ingredients and set aside.
3. In a small bowl, whisk together flour, baking powder and salt and set aside.

4. In a large mixing bowl, combine sugar and lemon zest. Add butter and beat until light and fluffy. Add eggs, vanilla and milk.
5. Add flour mixture and mix just until combine. Stir in blueberries and spread batter evenly into bread maker pan.
6. Top with crumb topping; select Sweet bread, light color crust, and press Start.
7. When done cool on a wire rack for 15 minutes and serve warm.

Nutrition Info: Calories: 462, Sodium: 332 mg, Dietary Fiber: 1 g, Fat: 32.1 g, Carbs: 41.8 g, Protein: 4 g.

Honey Nut Bread

Servings: 8
Cooking Time: 3 Hours And 25 Minutes
Ingredients:
- Eggs – 2
- Cottage cheese – 2/3 cup
- Milk – ½ cup
- Butter – ¼ cup
- Honey – 2 tbsp.
- All-purpose flour – 4 cups
- Instant yeast – 1 tbsp.
- Salt – 1 tsp.
- Candied nuts – ¾ cups, chopped

Directions:
1. Add everything, except nuts to your bread machine according to manufacturer recommendation.
2. Select Basic and choose Light crust type. Press Start.
3. Add the nuts when the machine beeps.
4. Remove the bread when ready.
5. Cool, slice, and serve.

Nutrition Info: (Per Serving): Calories: 422; Total Fat: 13.9 g; Saturated Fat: 5.2 g; Carbohydrates: 59.8 g; Cholesterol: 59 mg; Fiber: 2.8 g; Calcium: 62 mg; Sodium: 450 mg; Protein: 13.7 g

Pumpkin Spice Cake

Servings: 12
Cooking Time: 2 Hours 50 Minutes
Ingredients:
- 1 cup sugar

- 1 cup canned pumpkin
- 1/3 cup vegetable oil
- 1 teaspoon vanilla extract
- 2 eggs
- 1 1/2 cups all-purpose flour
- 2 teaspoons baking powder
- 1/4 teaspoon salt
- 1 teaspoon ground cinnamon
- 1/4 teaspoon ground nutmeg
- 1/8 teaspoon ground cloves
- Shortening, for greasing pan

Directions:
1. Grease bread maker pan and kneading blade generously with shortening.
2. Add all ingredients to the bread maker pan in the order listed above.
3. Select Rapid cycle and press Start.
4. Open the lid three minutes into the cycle and carefully scrape down sides of pan with a rubber spatula; close lid to continue cycle.
5. Cool baked cake for 10 minutes on a wire rack before slicing.

Nutrition Info: Calories: 195, Sodium: 64 mg, Dietary Fiber: 1.3 g, Fat: 7.1 g, Carbs: 31.2 g, Protein: 2.8 g.

Honey Wheat Bread

Servings: 1 Loaf
Ingredients:
- 16 slice bread (2 pounds)
- 1⅔ cups boiling water
- ¼ cup + 4 teaspoons cracked wheat
- ¼ cup + 4 teaspoons unsalted butter, melted
- ¼ cup honey
- 2 teaspoons table salt
- 1⅓ cups whole-wheat flour
- 2⅔ cups white bread flour
- 2½ teaspoons bread machine yeast
- 12 slice bread (1½ pounds)
- 1¼ cups boiling water
- ¼ cup cracked wheat
- ¼ cup unsalted butter, melted
- 3 tablespoons honey
- 1½ teaspoons table salt
- 1 cup whole-wheat flour

- 2 cups white bread flour
- 2 teaspoons bread machine yeast

Directions:

1. Choose the size of loaf you would like to make and measure your ingredients.
2. Add the boiling water and cracked wheat to the bread pan; set aside for 25–30 minutes for the wheat to soften.
3. Add the other ingredients to the bread pan in the order listed above.
4. Place the pan in the bread machine and close the lid.
5. Turn on the bread maker. Select the White/Basic setting, then the loaf size, and finally the crust color. Start the cycle.
6. When the cycle is finished and the bread is baked, carefully remove the pan from the machine. Use a potholder as the handle will be very hot. Let rest for a few minutes.
7. Remove the bread from the pan and allow to cool on a wire rack for at least 10 minutes before slicing.

Nutrition Info: (Per Serving):Calories 168, fat 4.3 g, carbs 31.3 g, sodium 296 mg, protein 4.1 g

Savory Bread Maker Rolls

Servings: 24
Cooking Time: 2 Hours 10 Mins
Ingredients:

- 1 cup warm milk, 70° to 80°F
- 1/2 cup butter, softened
- 1/4 cup sugar
- 2 eggs
- 1 1/2 teaspoons salt
- 4 cups bread flour
- 2 tablespoons herbes de Provence
- 2 1/4 teaspoons active dry yeast
- Flour, for surface

Directions:

1. Add all ingredients in the order listed above to the bread maker pan, reserving yeast.
2. Make a well in the flour; add yeast to the hole.
3. Select Dough setting; when Dough cycle is completed, turn dough out onto a lightly floured surface.

4. Divide dough into 24 portions and shape into balls.
5. Place rolls in a greased 13-by-9-inch baking pan.
6. Cover and let rise in a warm place for 30-45 minutes; preheat an oven to 350°F.
7. Bake for 13-16 minutes or until golden brown and serve warm.

Nutrition Info: Calories: 129, Sodium: 185 mg, Dietary Fiber: 0.6 g, Fat: 4.6 g, Carbs: 18.7 g, Protein: 3.1 g.

100% Whole Wheat Bread

Servings: 1 Loaf
Ingredients:

- 16 slice bread (2 pounds)
- 1¼ cups lukewarm water
- 2 tablespoons vegetable oil or olive oil
- ¼ cup honey or maple syrup
- 1½ teaspoons table salt
- 3½ cups whole wheat flour
- ¼ cup sesame, sunflower, or flax seeds (optional)
- 1½ teaspoons bread machine yeast
- 12 slice bread (1½ pounds)
- 1 cup lukewarm water
- 1½ tablespoons vegetable oil or olive oil
- 3 tablespoons honey or maple syrup
- 1 teaspoon table salt
- 2 ⅔ cups whole wheat flour
- 3 tablespoons sesame, sunflower, or flax seeds (optional)
- 1 teaspoon bread machine yeast

Directions:

1. Choose the size of loaf you would like to make and measure your ingredients.
2. Add the ingredients to the bread pan in the order listed above.
3. Place the pan in the bread machine and close the lid.
4. Turn on the bread maker. Select the Whole Wheat/Wholegrain setting, then the loaf size, and finally the crust color. Start the cycle.
5. When the cycle is finished, and the bread is baked, carefully remove the pan from the machine. Use a potholder as the handle will be very hot. Let rest for a few minutes.

6. Remove the bread from the pan and allow to cool on a wire rack for at least 10 minutes before slicing.

Nutrition Info: (Per Serving):Calories 147, fat 5.8 g, carbs 22.1 g, sodium 138 mg, protein 3.4 g

German Butter Cake

Servings: 12 - 16
Cooking Time: 2 Hour 25 Minutes
Ingredients:
- 2 teaspoons active dry yeast
- 1/4 cup sugar
- 2 1/4 cups all-purpose flour
- 1 teaspoon salt
- 7/8 cup whole milk, lukewarm
- 1 egg yolk
- 1 tablespoon butter, softened
- For the topping:
- 3 tablespoons butter, cold
- 1/2 cup almonds, sliced
- 1/3 cup sugar

Directions:
1. Add all of the dough ingredients to the bread maker pan.
2. Press Dough cycle and Start.
3. Grease a 10-inch springform pan; when the dough cycle is finished, pat the dough into the pan.
4. Prepare the topping by cutting the butter into - inch squares and place them sporadically over the surface of the dough, slightly pushing each into the dough.
5. Sprinkle with almond slices, then sprinkle evenly with sugar.
6. Cover with a towel and let stand in a warm place for 30 minutes.
7. Preheat an oven to 375F.
8. Bake for 20 to 25 minutes or until golden brown.
9. Let cool 10 minutes in pan on cooling rack and serve warm!

Nutrition Info: Calories: 226, Sodium: 228 mg, Dietary Fiber: 1 g, Fat: 9.1 g, Carbs: 29.8 g, Protein: 7.1 g.

Chocolate Marble Cake

Servings: 12 - 16

Cooking Time: 3 Hours 45 Minutes
Ingredients:
- 1 1/2 cups water
- 1 1/2 teaspoons vanilla extract
- 1 1/2 teaspoons salt
- 3 1/2 cups bread flour
- 1 1/2 teaspoons instant yeast
- 1 cup semi-sweet chocolate chips

Directions:
1. Set the chocolate chips aside and add the other ingredients to the pan of your bread maker.
2. Program the machine for Sweet bread and press Start.
3. Check the dough after 10 to 15 minutes of kneading; you should have a smooth ball, soft but not sticky.
4. Add the chocolate chips about 3 minutes before the end of the second kneading cycle.
5. Once baked, remove with a rubber spatula and allow to cool on a rack before serving.

Nutrition Info: Calories: 172, Sodium: 218 mg, Dietary Fiber: 1.6 g, Fat: 4.3 g, Carbs: 30.1 g, Protein: 3 g.

Classic White Sandwich Bread

Servings: 1 Loaf
Ingredients:
- 16 slice bread (2 pounds)
- 1 cup water, lukewarm between 80 and 90^{0}F
- 2 tablespoons unsalted butter, melted
- 1 teaspoon table salt
- 1/4 cup sugar
- 2 egg whites or 1 egg, beaten
- 3 cups white bread flour
- 1 1/2 teaspoons bread machine yeast
- 12 slice bread (1 ½ pounds)
- 3/4 cup water, lukewarm between 80 and 90^{0}F
- 1 1/2 tablespoons unsalted butter, melted
- 3/4 teaspoon table salt
- 1 ½ ounces sugar
- 2 egg whites or 1 egg, beaten
- 2 1/4 cups white bread flour
- 1 1/8 teaspoons bread machine yeast

Directions:

1. Choose the size of loaf you would like to make and measure your ingredients.
2. Add the ingredients to the bread pan in the order listed above.
3. Place the pan in the bread machine and close the lid.
4. Turn on the bread maker. Select the White/Basic setting, then the loaf size, and finally the crust color. Start the cycle.
5. When the cycle is finished and the bread is baked, carefully remove the pan from the machine. Use a potholder as the handle will be very hot. Let rest for a few minutes.
6. Remove the bread from the pan and allow to cool on a wire rack for at least 10 minutes before slicing.

Nutrition Info: (Per Serving):Calories 126, fat 2.3 g, carbs 23 g, sodium 137 mg, protein 4 g

Classic Dark Bread

Servings: 1 Loaf

Ingredients:
- 16 slice bread (2 pounds)
- 1¼ cups lukewarm water
- 2 tablespoons unsalted butter, melted
- ½ cup molasses
- ½ teaspoon table salt
- 1 cup rye flour
- 2½ cups white bread flour
- 2 tablespoons unsweetened cocoa powder
- Pinch ground nutmeg
- 2¼ teaspoons bread machine yeast
- 12 slice bread (1½ pounds)
- 1 cup lukewarm water
- 1½ tablespoons unsalted butter, melted
- ⅓ cup molasses
- ⅓ teaspoon table salt
- ¾ cup rye flour
- 2 cups white bread flour
- 1½ tablespoons unsweetened cocoa powder
- Pinch ground nutmeg
- 1⅔ teaspoons bread machine yeast

Directions:
1. Choose the size of loaf you would like to make and measure your ingredients.

2. Add the ingredients to the bread pan in the order listed above.
3. Place the pan in the bread machine and close the lid.
4. Turn on the bread maker. Select the White/Basic setting, then the loaf size, and finally the crust color. Start the cycle.
5. When the cycle is finished and the bread is baked, carefully remove the pan from the machine. Use a potholder as the handle will be very hot. Let rest for a few minutes.
6. Remove the bread from the pan and allow to cool on a wire rack for at least 10 minutes before slicing.

Nutrition Info: (Per Serving):Calories 143, fat 2.3 g, carbs 28.6 g, sodium 237 mg, protein 3.8 g

Cinnamon Rolls

Servings: 12 Rolls
Cooking Time: 2 H.

Ingredients:
- For the cinnamon roll dough:
- 1 cup milk
- 1 large egg
- 4 Tbsp butter
- 3⅓ cups bread flour
- 3 Tbsp sugar
- ½ tsp salt
- 2 tsp active dry yeast
- For the filling:
- ¼ cup butter, melted
- ¼ cup sugar
- 2 tsp cinnamon
- ½ tsp nutmeg
- ⅓ cup nuts, chopped and toasted
- For the icing:
- 1 cup powdered sugar
- 1 - 2 Tbsp milk
- ½ tsp vanilla

Directions:
1. Add each ingredient to the bread machine in the order and at the temperature recommended by your bread machine manufacturer.
2. Select the dough cycle and press start.

3. When it's done, transfer the dough onto a floured surface.

4. Knead it for 1 minute, then let it rest for the next 15 minutes.

5. Roll out a rectangle. Spread ¼ cup of melted butter over the dough.

6. Sprinkle the dough with cinnamon, ¼ cup sugar, nutmeg, and nuts.

7. Roll the dough, beginning from a long side. Seal the edges and form an evenly shaped roll. Cut it into 1-inch pieces.

8. Put them on a greased baking pan.

9. Cover with towel and leave for 45 minutes to rise.

10. Bake at 375°F in a preheated oven for 20-25 minutes.

11. Remove from the oven. Cool for 10 minutes.

12. Mix the icing ingredients in a bowl. Adjust with sugar or milk to desired thickness.

13. Cover the rolls with icing and serve.

Garlic Cheese Pull-apart Rolls

Servings: 12 - 24
Cooking Time: 3 Hours
Ingredients:

- 1 cup water
- 3 cups bread flour
- 1 1/2 teaspoons salt
- 1-1/2 tablespoons butter
- 3 tablespoons sugar
- 2 tablespoons nonfat dry milk powder
- 2 teaspoons yeast
- For the topping:
- 1/4 cup butter, melted
- 1 garlic clove, crushed
- 2 tablespoons parmesan cheese, plus more if needed
- Flour, for surface

Directions:

1. Place first 6 ingredients in bread maker pan in order listed.

2. Make a well in the flour; pour the yeast into the hole.

3. Select Dough cycle, press Start.

4. Turn finished dough onto a floured countertop.

5. Gently roll and stretch dough into a 24-inch rope.

6. Grease a 13-by-9-inch baking sheet.

7. Divide dough into 24 pieces with a sharp knife and shape into balls; place on prepared pan. Combine butter and garlic in a small mixing bowl and pour over rolls.

8. Sprinkle rolls evenly with parmesan cheese.

9. Cover and let rise for 30-45 minutes until doubled.

10. Bake at 375°F for 10 to 15 minutes or until golden brown.

11. Remove from oven, pull apart, and serve warm.

Nutrition Info: Calories: 109, Sodium: 210 mg, Dietary Fiber: 0.6 g, Fat: 3.5 g, Carbs: 16.7 g, Protein: 2.6 g.

10 Minute Rosemary Bread

Servings: 12
Cooking Time: 2 Hours
Ingredients:

- 1 cup warm water, about 105°F
- 2 tablespoons butter, softened
- 1 egg
- 3 cups all-purpose flour
- 1/4 cup whole wheat flour
- 1/3 cup sugar
- 1 teaspoon salt
- 3 teaspoons bread maker yeast
- 2 tablespoons rosemary, freshly chopped
- For the topping:
- 1 egg, room temperature
- 1 teaspoon milk, room temperature
- Garlic powder
- Sea salt

Directions:

1. Place all of the ingredients in the bread maker pan in the order listed above.

2. Select Dough cycle.

3. When dough is kneaded, place on parchment paper on a flat surface and roll into two loaves; set aside and allow to rise for 30 minutes.

4. Preheat a pizza stone in an oven on 375°F for 30 minutes.

5. For the topping, add the egg and milk to a small mixing bowl and whisk to create an egg wash. Baste the formed loaves and sprinkle evenly with garlic powder and sea salt.

6. Allow to rise for 40 minutes, lightly covered, in a warm area.
7. Bake for 15 to 18 minutes or until golden brown. Serve warm.
Nutrition Info: Calories: 176, Sodium: 220 mg, Dietary Fiber: 1.5 g, Fat: 3.1 g, Carbs: 32 g, Protein: 5 g.

Apple Pecan Cinnamon Rolls

Servings: 12 Rolls
Cooking Time: 3 H.
Ingredients:
- 1 cup warm milk (70ºF to 80ºF)
- 2 large eggs
- ⅓ cup butter, melted
- ½ cup sugar
- 1 tsp salt
- 4½ cups bread flour
- 2½ tsp bread machine yeast
- For the filling:
- 3 Tbsp butter, melted
- 1 cup finely chopped peeled apples
- ¾ cup packed brown sugar
- ⅓ cup chopped pecans
- 2½ tsp ground cinnamon
- For the icing:
- 1½ cup confectioners sugar
- ⅜ cup cream cheese, softened
- ¼ cup butter, softened
- ½ tsp vanilla extract
- ⅛ tsp salt drained

Directions:
1. Add each ingredient for the dough to the bread machine in order stipulated by the manufacturer.
2. Set to dough cycle and press start.
3. When cycle has completed, place the dough onto a well-floured surface. Roll it into a rectangle. Brush it with butter.
4. Mix the brown sugar, apples, pecans, and cinnamon in a bowl. Spread over the dough evenly.
5. Beginning from the long side, roll the dough. Cut it into 1¾-inch slices.
6. Transfer them onto a greased baking dish. Cover and let rise for 30 minutes.

7. Bake at 325°F in a preheated oven for 25-30 minutes.
8. Meanwhile, mix all the icing ingredients in a bowl.
9. Take out the rolls and let them cool
10. Cover warm rolls with the glaze and serve.

Honey Pound Cake

Servings: 12 - 16
Cooking Time: 2 Hours 50 Minutes
Ingredients:
- 1 cup butter, unsalted
- 1/4 cup honey
- 2 tablespoons whole milk
- 4 eggs, beaten
- 1 cup sugar
- 2 cups flour

Directions:
1. Bring the butter to room temperature and cut into 1/2-inch cubes.
2. Add the ingredients to the bread machine in the order listed (butter, honey, milk, eggs, sugar, flour).
3. Press Sweet bread setting, light crust color, and press Start.
4. Take the cake out of the bread pan using a rubber spatula, as soon as it's finished. Cool on a rack and serve with your favorite fruit.
Nutrition Info: Calories: 117, Sodium: 183 mg, Dietary Fiber: 0.3 g, Fat: 6.9 g, Carbs: 12.3 g, Protein: 1.9 g.

Apple Raisin Nut Cake

Servings: 10
Cooking Time: 45 Minutes
Ingredients:
- 2 large eggs, lightly beaten
- 1/4 cup milk
- 1/3 cup butter, melted
- 1 1/2 cups all-purpose flour
- 3 teaspoons baking powder
- 1/4 cup sugar
- 1/4 teaspoon salt
- 1 teaspoon cinnamon
- 1 teaspoon pure vanilla extract
- Add after the kneading process:

- 1 small apple, peeled and roughly chopped
- 1/4 cup raisins
- 1/4 cup walnuts, chopped
- 1 teaspoon all-purpose flour

Directions:
1. Add ingredients in the order listed above.
2. Press Sweet cycle, light color crust, and Start.
3. Mix apples, raisins, walnuts, and flour together in a small mixing bowl. Add to dough after the kneading process.
4. Allow to cool on a cooling rack for 15 minutes before serving.

Nutrition Info: Calories: 204, Sodium: 121 mg, Dietary Fiber: 1.5 g, Fat: 9.4 g, Carbs: 26.9 g, Protein: 4.4 g.

Classic Whole Wheat Bread

Servings: 1 Loaf

Ingredients:
- 16 slice bread (2 pounds)
- 1 cup lukewarm water
- ½ cup unsalted butter, melted
- 2 eggs, at room temperature
- 2 teaspoons table salt
- ¼ cup sugar
- 1½ cups whole-wheat flour
- 2½ cups white bread flour
- 2¼ teaspoons bread machine yeast
- 12 slice bread (1½ pounds)
- ¾ cup lukewarm water
- ⅓ cup unsalted butter, melted
- 2 eggs, at room temperature
- 1½ teaspoons table salt
- 3 tablespoons sugar
- 1 cup whole-wheat flour
- 2 cups white bread flour
- 1⅔ teaspoons bread machine yeast

Directions:
1. Choose the size of loaf you would like to make and measure your ingredients.
2. Add the ingredients to the bread pan in the order listed above.
3. Place the pan in the bread machine and close the lid.

4. Turn on the bread maker. Select the Whole Wheat/ Wholegrain or White/Basic setting, wither one will work well for this recipe. Then select the loaf size, and finally the crust color. Start the cycle.
5. When the cycle is finished and the bread is baked, carefully remove the pan from the machine. Use a potholder as the handle will be very hot. Let rest for a few minutes.
6. Remove the bread from the pan and allow to cool on a wire rack for at least 10 minutes before slicing.

Nutrition Info: (Per Serving):Calories 176, fat 5.3 g, carbs 24.2 g, sodium 294 mg, protein 5.2 g

Onion Loaf

Servings: 12
Cooking Time: 3 Hours 40 Minutes

Ingredients:
- 1 tablespoon butter
- 2 medium onions, sliced
- 1 cup water
- 1 tablespoon olive or vegetable oil
- 3 cups bread flour
- 2 tablespoons sugar
- 1 teaspoon salt
- 1 1/4 teaspoons bread machine or quick active dry yeast

Directions:
1. Preheat a large skillet to medium-low heat and add butter to melt. Add onions and cook for 10 to 15 minutes, stirring often, until onions are brown and caramelized; remove from heat.
2. Add remaining ingredients, except onions, to the bread maker pan in the order listed above.
3. Select the Basic cycle, medium crust color, and press Start.
4. Add 1/2 cup of the onions 5 to 10 minutes before the last kneading cycle ends.
5. Remove baked bread from pan and allow to cool on a cooling rack before serving.

Nutrition Info: Calories: 149, Sodium: 203 mg, Dietary Fiber: 1.3 g, Fat: 2.5 g, Carbs: 27.7 g, Protein: 3.7 g.

Parsley And Chive Pull-apart Rolls

Servings: 16
Cooking Time: 3 Hours
Ingredients:

- 1 cup buttermilk
- 6 tablespoons unsalted butter, cut into 6 pieces
- 3 2/3 cups all-purpose flour
- 2 1/4 teaspoons instant yeast
- 1/3 cup granulated sugar
- 1 teaspoon salt
- 3 large egg yolks
- 1/4 cup chives, chopped
- 1/4 cup parsley, chopped
- For the topping:
- 1/4 cup butter, melted

Directions:

1. Combine the buttermilk and the 6 tablespoons butter in a small saucepan and warm until the butter melts, stirring continuously. Add the packet of instant yeast and allow to stand for five minutes.
2. Mix the egg yolks with a fork and add to the above mixture and blend.
3. Combine the flour, sugar, salt and herbs.
4. Add first the wet then the dry ingredients to your bread machine.
5. Set on Dough cycle and press Start.
6. Lightly grease a 9-by-13-inch glass baking dish.
7. Turn the dough out onto a clean work surface and press down gently. If the dough is too sticky add a little flour to the work surface. Using a bench scraper or a chef's knife, divide the dough into 16 equal pieces
8. Work one piece of dough at a time into a ball; keep the others covered with plastic wrap until ready to bake.
9. Cover the entire baking dish with plastic wrap and let the balls rise in a warm space, about 40 to 60 minutes.
10. Preheat an oven to 375°F and bake 20 to 25 minutes, or until lightly golden brown.
11. Remove from the oven and brush the tops with melted butter, serve warm.

Nutrition Info: Calories: 196, Sodium: 201 mg, Dietary Fiber: 0.9 g, Fat: 8.4 g, Carbs: 26.5 g, Protein: 3.8 g.

Apple Walnut Bread

Servings: 14 Slices
Cooking Time: 2 H. 30 Min.
Ingredients:

- ¾ cup unsweetened applesauce
- 4 cups apple juice
- 1 tsp salt
- 3 Tbsp butter
- 1 large egg
- 4 cups bread flour
- ¼ cup brown sugar, packed
- 1¼ tsp cinnamon
- ½ tsp baking soda
- 2 tsp active dry yeast
- ½ cup chopped walnuts
- ½ cup chopped dried cranberries

Directions:

1. Add each ingredient to the bread machine in the order and at the temperature recommended by your bread machine manufacturer.
2. Close the lid, select the basic bread, medium crust setting on your bread machine, and press start.
3. When the bread machine has finished baking, remove the bread and put it on a cooling rack.

Whole-wheat Bread

Servings: 8
Cooking Time: 3 Hours And 48 Minutes
Ingredients:

- Water - ¾ cup
- Melted butter - 1½ tbsp., cooled
- Honey - 1½ tbsp.
- Salt - ¾ tsp.
- Whole-wheat bread flour - 2 cups
- Bread machine or instant yeast - 1 tsp.

Directions:

1. Add the ingredients in the machine according to the manufacturer's instructions.
2. Press Whole-Wheat/Whole-Grain bread, choose Light or Medium crust, and press Start.
3. When done, remove the bread from the machine and cool.
4. Slice and serve.

Nutrition Info: (Per Serving): Calories: 146; Total Fat: 3 g; Saturated Fat: 1 g; Carbohydrates: 27 g;

Cholesterol: 8 mg; Fiber: 1 g; Calcium: 14 mg; Sodium: 210 mg; Protein: 3 g

Blue Cheese Bread

Servings: 10 - 12
Cooking Time: 3 Hours
Ingredients:
- 3/4 cup warm water
- 1 large egg
- 1 teaspoon salt
- 3 cups bread flour
- 1 cup blue cheese, crumbled
- 2 tablespoons nonfat dry milk
- 2 tablespoons sugar
- 1 teaspoon bread machine yeast

Directions:
1. Add the ingredients to bread machine pan in the order listed above, (except yeast) ; be sure to add the cheese with the flour.
2. Make a well in the flour; pour the yeast into the hole.
3. Select Basic bread cycle, medium crust color, and press Start.
4. When finished, transfer to a cooling rack for 10 minutes and serve warm.
Nutrition Info: Calories: 171, Sodium: 266 mg, Dietary Fiber: 0.9 g, Fat: 3.9 g, Carbs: 26.8 g, Protein: 6.7 g.

Caramelized Onion Focaccia Bread

Servings: 4 – 6
Cooking Time: 3 Hours
Ingredients:
- 3/4 cup water
- 2 tablespoons olive oil
- 1 tablespoon sugar
- 1 teaspoon salt
- 2 cups flour
- 1 1/2 teaspoons yeast
- 3/4 cup mozzarella cheese, shredded
- 2 tablespoons parmesan cheese, shredded
- Onion topping:
- 3 tablespoons butter
- 2 medium onions
- 2 cloves garlic, minced

Directions:
1. Place all ingredients, except cheese and onion topping, in your bread maker in the order listed above.
2. Grease a large baking sheet.
3. Pat dough into a 12-inch circle on the pan; cover and let rise in warm place for about 30 minutes.
4. Melt butter in large frying pan over medium-low heat. Cook onions and garlic in butter 15 minutes, stirring often, until onions are caramelized.
5. Preheat an oven to 400°F.
6. Make deep depressions across the dough at 1-inch intervals with the handle of a wooden spoon.
7. Spread the onion topping over dough and sprinkle with cheeses.
8. Bake 15 to 20 minutes or until golden brown. Cut into wedges and serve warm.
Nutrition Info: Calories: 286, Sodium: 482 mg, Dietary Fiber: 2.2 g, Fat: 12 g, Carbs: 38.1 g, Protein: 6.8 g.

Garlic Basil Knots

Servings: 10
Cooking Time: 1 Hour 45 Minutes
Ingredients:
- 1 cup water
- 2 tablespoons butter, softened
- 1 egg, room temperature
- 3 1/4 cups all-purpose flour
- 1/4 cup sugar
- 1 teaspoon salt
- 3 teaspoons regular active dry yeast
- For the topping:
- 2 tablespoons butter, melted
- 2 cloves garlic, minced
- 3 fresh basil leaves, chopped fine
- Flour, for surface

Directions:
1. Add all dough ingredients in the bread machine in the order listed.
2. Select the Dough cycle and press Start.
3. Place parchment paper on a baking sheet and coat with cooking spray.
4. Flatten the dough onto a well-floured surface and cut into strips using a pizza cutter.

5. Tie each strip into a knot, making sure to keep them well-floured so they don't stick together. Place knots on the baking sheet and cover with a cloth; set in a warm place to rise for 30 minutes.

6. Preheat oven to 400°F and bake 9 to 12 minutes or until golden brown.

7. Serve warm!

Nutrition Info: Calories: 218, Sodium: 274 mg, Dietary Fiber: 1.4 g, Fat: 5.5 g, Carbs: 36.7 g, Protein: 5.3 g.

Sunflower And Flax Seed Bread

Servings: 15

Cooking Time: 3 Hours And 25 Minutes

Ingredients:
- Water – 1 1/3 cups
- Butter – 2 tbsp., softened
- Honey – 3 tbsp.
- Bread flour – 1 ½ cups
- Whole wheat bread flour – 1 1/3 cups
- Salt – 1 tsp.
- Active dry yeast – 1 tsp.
- Flax seeds – ½ cup
- Sunflower seeds – ½ cup

Directions:
1. Place everything (except sunflower seeds) in the bread machine according to machine recommendation.
2. Select Basic White cycle and press Start.
3. Add the seeds after the alert sounds.
4. Cool, slice, and serve.

Nutrition Info: (Per Serving): Calories: 140.3; Total Fat: 4.2 g; Saturated Fat: 1.2 g; Carbohydrates: 22.7 g; Cholesterol: 4.1 mg; Fiber: 3.1 g; Calcium: 19.8 mg; Sodium: 168.6 mg; Protein: 4.2 g

Basic Bulgur Bread

Servings: 1 Loaf

Ingredients:
- 16 slice bread (2 pounds)
- ½ cup lukewarm water
- ½ cup bulgur wheat
- 1⅓ cups lukewarm milk
- 1⅓ tablespoons unsalted butter, melted
- 1⅓ tablespoons sugar

- 1 teaspoon table salt
- 4 cups bread flour
- 2 teaspoons bread machine yeast
- 12 slice bread (1½ pounds)
- ⅓ cup lukewarm water
- ⅓ cup bulgur wheat
- 1 cup lukewarm milk
- 1 tablespoon unsalted butter, melted
- 1 tablespoon sugar
- ¾ teaspoon table salt
- 3 cups bread flour
- 1½ teaspoons bread machine yeast

Directions:
1. Choose the size of loaf you would like to make and measure your ingredients.
2. Add the water and bulgur wheat to the bread pan and set aside for 25–30 minutes for the bulgur wheat to soften.
3. Add the other ingredients to the bread pan in the order listed above.
4. Place the pan in the bread machine and close the lid.
5. Turn on the bread maker. Select the White/Basic setting, then the loaf size, and finally the crust color. Start the cycle.
6. When the cycle is finished and the bread is baked, carefully remove the pan from the machine. Use a potholder as the handle will be very hot. Let rest for a few minutes.
7. Remove the bread from the pan and allow to cool on a wire rack for at least 10 minutes before slicing.

Nutrition Info: (Per Serving):Calories 160, fat 2.6 g, carbs 28.7 g, sodium 163 mg, protein 5 g

Texas Roadhouse Rolls

Servings: 18 Rolls

Cooking Time: 20 Min.

Ingredients:
- ¼ cup warm water (80ºF - 90ºF
- 1 cup warm milk (80ºF -90ºF)
- 1 tsp salt
- 1½ Tbsp butter + more for brushing
- 1 egg
- ¼ cup sugar

- 3½ cups unbleached bread flour
- 1 envelope dry active yeast
- For Texas roadhouse cinnamon butter:
- ½ cup sweet, creamy salted butter, softened
- ⅓ cup confectioners' sugar
- 1 tsp ground cinnamon

Directions:

1. Add each ingredient to the bread machine in the order and at the temperature recommended by your bread machine manufacturer.
2. Select the dough cycle and press start.
3. Once cycle is done, transfer your dough onto a lightly floured surface.
4. Roll out the rectangle, fold it in half. Let it rest for 15 minutes.
5. Cut the roll into 18 squares. Transfer them onto a baking sheet.
6. Bake at 350°F in a preheated oven for 10-15 minutes.
7. Remove dough from the oven and brush the top with butter.
8. Beat the softened butter with a mixer to make it fluffy. Gradually add the sugar and cinnamon while blending. Mix well.
9. Take out the rolls, let them cool for 2-3 minutes.
10. Spread them with cinnamon butter on the top while they are warm.

Golden Turmeric Cardamom Bread

Servings: 12

Cooking Time: 3 Hours

Ingredients:

- 1 cup lukewarm water
- 1/3 cup lukewarm milk
- 3 tablespoons butter, unsalted
- 3 3/4 cups unbleached all-purpose flour
- 3 tablespoons sugar
- 1 1/2 teaspoons salt
- 2 tablespoons ground turmeric
- 1 tablespoon ground cardamom
- 1/2 teaspoon cayenne pepper
- 1 1/2 teaspoons active dry yeast

Directions:

1. Add liquid ingredients to the bread pan.
2. Measure and add dry ingredients (except yeast) to the bread pan.
3. Make a well in the center of the dry ingredients and add the yeast.
4. Snap the baking pan into the bread maker and close the lid.
5. Choose the Basic setting, preferred crust color and press Start.
6. When the loaf is done, remove the pan from the machine. After about 5 minutes, gently shake the pan to loosen the loaf and turn it out onto a rack to cool.

Nutrition Info: Calories: 183, Sodium: 316 mg, Dietary Fiber: 1.2 g, Fat: 3.3 g, Carbs: 33.3 g, Protein: 4.5 g.

SPICE, NUT & HERB BREAD

Cheese Herb Bread

Servings: 10
Cooking Time: 3 Hours 27 Minutes
Ingredients:
- Active dry yeast – 1 ¼ tsps.
- Dried oregano – 1 ¼ tsps.
- Fennel seed – 1 ¼ tsps.
- Dried basil – 1 ¼ tsps.
- Asiago cheese – 2/3 cup, grated
- Bread flour – 3 ¼ cups
- Sugar – 1 tbsp.
- Salt – ¾ tsp.
- Water – 1 cup.

Directions:
1. Add all ingredients to the bread machine. Select sweet bread setting then select light/medium crust and start. Once loaf is done, remove the loaf pan from the machine. Allow it to cool for 10 minutes. Slice and serve.

Healthy Basil Whole Wheat Bread

Servings: 10
Cooking Time: 2 Hours
Ingredients:
- Olive oil – 2 tbsps.
- Basil – 1 tbsp.
- Water – 1 1/3 cups
- Whole wheat flour – 4 cups
- Salt – 2 tsps.
- Sugar – 3 tbsps.
- Active dry yeast – 2 tsps.

Directions:
1. Add olive oil and water to the bread pan. Add remaining ingredients except for yeast to the bread pan. Make a small hole into the flour with your finger and add yeast to the hole. Make sure yeast will not be mixed with any liquids. Select whole wheat setting then select light/medium crust and start. Once loaf is done, remove the loaf pan from the machine. Allow it to cool for 5 minutes. Slice and serve.

Pecan Raisin Bread

Servings: 1 Loaf

Cooking Time: 10 Minutes Plus Fermenting Time
Ingredients:
- 1 cup plus 2 Tbsp water (70°F to 80°F)
- 8 tsp butter
- 1 egg
- 6 Tbsp sugar
- ¼ cup nonfat dry milk powder
- 1 tsp salt
- 4 cups bread flour
- 1 Tbsp active dry yeast
- 1 cup finely chopped pecans
- 1 cup raisins

Directions:
1. Preparing the Ingredients
2. Add each ingredient to the bread machine except the pecans and raisins in the order and at the temperature recommended by your bread machine manufacturer.
3. Select the Bake cycle
4. Close the lid, select the basic bread, medium crust setting on your bread machine, and press start.
5. Just before the final kneading, add the pecans and raisins.
6. When the bread machine has finished baking, remove the bread and put it on a cooling rack.

Flaxseed Honey Bread

Servings: 1 Loaf
Cooking Time: 10 Minutes
Ingredients:
- 12 slices bread (1½ pounds)
- 1⅛ cups milk, at 80°F to 90°F
- 1½ tablespoons melted butter, cooled
- 1½ tablespoons honey
- 1 teaspoon salt
- ¼ cup flaxseed
- 3 cups white bread flour
- 1¼ teaspoons bread machine or instant yeast

Directions:
1. Preparing the Ingredients.
2. Choose the size of loaf of your preference and then measure the ingredients.
3. Add all of the ingredients mentioned previously in the list.

4.   Close the lid after placing the pan in the bread machine.
5.   Select the Bake cycle.
6.   Turn on the bread machine. Select the White/Basic setting, select the loaf size, and the crust color. Press start.
7.   When the cycle is finished, carefully remove the pan from the bread maker and let it rest.
8.   Remove the bread from the pan, put in a wire rack to Cool about 5 minutes. Slice

Dilly Onion Bread

Servings: 14 Slices
Cooking Time: 3 H. 5 Min.

Ingredients:
- ¾ cup water (70°F to 80°F)
- 1 Tbsp butter, softened
- 2 Tbsp sugar
- 3 Tbsp dried minced onion
- 2 Tbsp dried parsley flakes
- 1 Tbsp dill weed
- 1 tsp salt
- 1 garlic clove, minced
- 2 cups bread flour
- ⅓ cup whole wheat flour
- 1 Tbsp nonfat dry milk powder
- 2 tsp active dry yeast serving

Directions:
1.   Add each ingredient to the bread machine in the order and at the temperature recommended by your bread machine manufacturer.
2.   Close the lid, select the basic bread, medium crust setting on your bread machine and press start.
3.   When the bread machine has finished baking, remove the bread and put it on a cooling rack.

French Herb Bread

Servings: 10
Cooking Time: 3 Hours 30 Minutes

Ingredients:
- All-purpose flour – 3 cups
- Instant dry yeast – 2 ½ tsps.
- Sugar – 3 tbsps.
- Garlic powder – ½ tsp.
- Sea salt – 1 ½ tsps.

- Warm water – 1 cup.
- Dried oregano – ½ tsp.
- Dried basil – ½ tsp.
- Dried ground thyme – 1/8 tsp.
- Dried rosemary – 1 tsp.
- Olive oil – 3 tbsps.

Directions:
1.   In a small bowl, mix together dried herbs and olive oil and set aside. Add water salt, sugar, yeast, oil herb mixture, and flour into the bread machine pan. Select French bread setting then select light crust and start. Once loaf is done, remove the loaf pan from the machine. Allow it to cool for 10 minutes. Slice and serve.

Pumpkin Cinnamon Bread

Servings: 14 Slices
Cooking Time: 3 H.

Ingredients:
- 1 cup sugar
- 1 cup canned pumpkin
- ⅓ cup vegetable oil
- 1 tsp vanilla
- 2 eggs
- 1½ cups all-purpose bread flour
- 2 tsp baking powder
- ¼ tsp salt
- 1 tsp ground cinnamon
- ¼ tsp ground nutmeg
- ⅛ tsp ground cloves

Directions:
1.   Add each ingredient to the bread machine in the order and at the temperature recommended by your bread machine manufacturer.
2.   Close the lid, select the quick, medium crust setting on your bread machine and press start.
3.   When the bread machine has finished baking, remove the bread and put it on a cooling rack.

Almond Milk Bread

Servings: 1 Loaf

Ingredients:
- 16 slice bread (2 pounds)
- 1 cup lukewarm milk
- 2 eggs, at room temperature

- 2⅔ tablespoons butter, melted and cooled
- ⅓ cup sugar
- 1 teaspoon table salt
- 2⅓ teaspoons lemon zest
- 4 cups white bread flour
- 2¼ teaspoons bread machine yeast
- ½ cup slivered almonds, chopped
- ½ cup golden raisins, chopped
- 12 slice bread (1½ pounds)
- ¾ cup lukewarm milk
- 2 eggs, at room temperature
- 2 tablespoons butter, melted and cooled
- ¼ cup sugar
- 1 teaspoon table salt
- 2 teaspoons lemon zest
- 3 cups white bread flour
- 2 teaspoons bread machine yeast
- ⅓ cup slivered almonds, chopped
- ⅓ cup golden raisins, chopped

Directions:

1. Choose the size of loaf you would like to make and measure your ingredients.
2. Add all of the ingredients except for the raisins and almonds to the bread pan in the order listed above.
3. Place the pan in the bread machine and close the lid.
4. Turn on the bread maker. Select the White/Basic or Fruit/Nut (if your machine has this setting) setting, then the loaf size, and finally the crust color. Start the cycle.
5. When the machine signals to add ingredients, add the raisins and almonds. (Some machines have a fruit/nut hopper where you can add the raisins and almonds when you start the machine. The machine will automatically add them to the dough during the baking process.)
6. When the cycle is finished and the bread is baked, carefully remove the pan from the machine. Use a potholder as the handle will be very hot. Let rest for a few minutes.
7. Remove the bread from the pan and allow to cool on a wire rack for at least 10 minutes before slicing.

Nutrition Info: (Per Serving):Calories 193, fat 4.6 g, carbs 29.4 g, sodium 214 mg, protein 5.7 g

Semolina Bread

Servings: 6 Pcs
Cooking Time: One Hour
Ingredients:

- Almond fine flour, one cup
- Semolina flour, one cup
- Yeast, one teaspoon
- An egg
- Salt, one teaspoon
- Stevia powder, two teaspoons
- Olive oil extra virgin, two teaspoons
- Water warm, one cup
- Sesame seeds, two teaspoons

Directions:

1. Get a mixing container and combine the almond flour, semolina flour, salt, and stevia powder.
2. In another mixing container, combine the egg
3. extra virgin olive oil, and warm water.
4. By instructions on your machine's manual, pour the ingredients in the bread pan and follow how to mix in the yeast.
5. Put the bread pan in the machine, select the basic bread setting
6. together with the bread size and crust type, if available, then press start once you have closed the machine's lid.
7. When the bread is ready, open the lid and spread the sesame seeds at the top and close for a few minutes.
8. By using oven mitts, remove the pan from the machine. Use a stainless spatula to extract the pan's bread and turn the pan upside down on a metallic rack where the bread will cool off before slicing it.

Nutrition Info: Calories: 100;Carbohydrates: 2.8g;Protein: 5g;Fat: 14g

Italian Pine Nut Bread

Servings: 10
Cooking Time: 3 Hours 30 Minutes
Ingredients:

- Water – 1 cup+ 2 tbsps.
- Bread flour – 3 cups.
- Sugar – 2 tbsps.
- Salt – 1 tsp.

- Active dry yeast – 1 ¼ tsps.
- Basil pesto – 1/3 cup.
- Flour – 2 tbsps.
- Pine nuts – 1/3 cup.

Directions:

1. In a small bowl, mix basil pesto and flour until well blended. Add pine nuts and stir well. Add water, bread flour, sugar, salt, and yeast into the bread machine pan. Select basic setting then select medium crust and press start. Add basil pesto mixture just before the final kneading cycle. Once loaf is done, remove the loaf pan from the machine. Allow it to cool for 10 minutes. Slice and serve.

Herb And Parmesan Bread

Servings: 10
Cooking Time: 3 Hours And 25 Minutes
Ingredients:

- Lukewarm water – 1 1/3 cups
- Oil – 2 tbsp.
- Garlic – cloves, crushed
- Fresh herbs – 3 tbsp., chopped (oregano, chives, basil, and rosemary)
- Bread flour – 4 cups
- Salt – 1 tsp.
- Sugar – 1 tbsp.
- Parmesan cheese – 4 tbsp., grated
- Active dry yeast – 2 ¼ tsp.

Directions:

1. Add everything according to bread machine recommendations.
2. Select Basic cycle and Medium crust.
3. When done, remove the bread.
4. Cool, slice, and serve.

Nutrition Info: (Per Serving): Calories: 105; Total Fat: 5 g; Saturated Fat: 1 g; Carbohydrates: 14 g; Cholesterol: 2 mg; Fiber: 2 g; Calcium: 94 mg; Sodium: 412 mg; Protein: 3 g

Turmeric Bread

Servings: 14 Slices
Cooking Time: 3 H.
Ingredients:

- 1 tsp dried yeast
- 4 cups strong white flour

- 1 tsp turmeric powder
- 2 tsp beetroot powder
- 2 Tbsp olive oil
- 1.5 tsp salt
- 1 tsp chili flakes
- 1⅜ water

Directions:

1. Add each ingredient to the bread machine in the order and at the temperature recommended by your bread machine manufacturer.
2. Close the lid, select the basic bread, medium crust setting on your bread machine and press start.
3. When the bread machine has finished baking, remove the bread and put it on a cooling rack.

Cardamom Honey Bread

Servings: 1 Loaf
Cooking Time: 10 Minutes
Ingredients:

- 16 slices bread (2 pounds)
- 1⅛ cups lukewarm milk
- 1 egg, at room temperature
- 2 teaspoons unsalted butter, melted
- ¼ cup honey
- 1⅓ teaspoons table salt
- 4 cups white bread flour
- 1⅓ teaspoons ground cardamom
- 1⅔ teaspoons bread machine yeast

Directions:

1. Preparing the Ingredients.
2. Choose the size of loaf of your preference and then measure the ingredients.
3. Add all of the ingredients mentioned previously in the list.
4. Close the lid after placing the pan in the bread machine.
5. Select the Bake cycle
6. Turn on the bread machine. Select the White/Basic setting, select the loaf size, and the crust color. Press start.
7. When the cycle is finished, carefully remove the pan from the bread maker and let it rest.
8. Remove the bread from the pan, put in a wire rack to Cool about 10 minutes. Slice

Quinoa Whole-wheat Bread

Servings: 1 Loaf
Cooking Time: 10 Minutes
Ingredients:
- 12 slice bread (1½ pounds)
- 1 cup milk, at 80°F to 90°F
- ⅔ cup cooked quinoa, cooled
- ¼ cup melted butter, cooled
- 1 tablespoon sugar
- 1 teaspoon salt
- ¼ cup quick oats
- ¾ cup whole-wheat flour
- 1½ cups white bread flour
- 1½ teaspoons bread machine or instant yeast

Directions:
1. Preparing the Ingredients.
2. Choose the size of loaf of your preference and then measure the ingredients.
3. Add all of the ingredients mentioned previously in the list.
4. Close the lid after placing the pan in the bread machine.
5. Select the Bake cycle
6. Turn on the bread machine. Select the White/Basic setting, select the loaf size, and the crust color. Press start.
7. When the cycle is finished, carefully remove the pan from the bread maker and let it rest.
8. Remove the bread from the pan, put in a wire rack to Cool about 5 minutes. Slice

Rosemary Garlic Dinner Rolls

Servings: 10 Pcs
Cooking Time: 30 Minutes
Ingredients:
- ½ teaspoon baking powder
- 1/3 cup ground flax seed
- 1 cup mozzarella cheese, shredded
- 1 cup almond flour
- One teaspoon rosemary, minced
- A pinch of salt
- 1 oz. cream cheese
- One egg
- beaten
- One tablespoon butter

- One teaspoon garlic, minced

Directions:
1. Add all ingredients to the Bread Machine.
2. Select Dough setting. When the time is over, transfer the dough to the floured surface. Shape it into a ball.
3. Roll the dough until it becomes a log and slice into six slices. Place on a greased baking sheet.
4. Combine rosemary, garlic, and butter in a bowl and mix—brush half of this over the biscuits.
5. Set the heat of the oven to 400F and bake for 15 minutes.
6. Brush with the remaining mixture and add salt before serving.

Nutrition Info: Calories: 168 Cal;Fat: 12.9g;Carbohydrates: 5.4g;Protein: 10.3g

Raisin Seed Bread

Servings: 1 Loaf
Cooking Time: 10 Minutes
Ingredients:
- 12 slice bread (1½ pounds)
- 1 cup plus 2 tablespoons milk, at 80°F to 90°F
- 1½ tablespoons melted butter, cooled
- 1½ tablespoons honey
- ¾ teaspoon salt
- 3 tablespoons flaxseed
- 3 tablespoons sesame seeds
- 1¼ cups whole-wheat flour
- 1¾ cups white bread flour
- 1¾ teaspoons bread machine or instant yeast
- ⅓ cup raisins
-

Directions:
1. Preparing the Ingredients.
2. Choose the size of loaf of your preference and then measure the ingredients.
3. Add all of the ingredients mentioned previously in the list except the raisins.
4. Close the lid after placing the pan in the bread machine.
5. Select the Bake cycle
6. Program the machine for Basic/White bread, select light or medium crust, and press Start.

7. Add the raisins when the bread machine signals, or place the raisins in the raisin/nut hopper and let the machine add them.
8. When the cycle is finished, carefully remove the pan from the bread maker and let it rest.
9. Remove the bread from the pan, put in a wire rack to Cool about 5 minutes. Slice

Sesame French Bread

Servings: 14 Slices
Cooking Time: 3 H. 15 Min.
Ingredients:

- ⅞ cup water
- 1 Tbsp butter, softened
- 3 cups bread flour
- 2 tsp sugar
- 1 tsp salt
- 2 tsp yeast
- 2 Tbsp sesame seeds toasted

Directions:
1. Add each ingredient to the bread machine in the order and at the temperature recommended by your bread machine manufacturer.
2. Close the lid, select the French bread, medium crust setting on your bread machine and press start.
3. When the bread machine has finished baking, remove the bread and put it on a cooling rack.

Onion Bacon Bread

Servings: 22 Slices
Cooking Time: 1 Hour
Ingredients:

- 1 ½ cups lukewarm water (80 degrees F)
- Two tablespoons sugar
- Three teaspoons active dry yeast
- 4 ½ cups wheat flour
- One whole egg
- Two teaspoons kosher salt
- One tablespoon olive oil
- Three small onions, chopped and lightly toasted
- 1 cup bacon, chopped

Directions:
1. Prepare all of the ingredients for your bread and measuring means (a cup, a spoon, kitchen scales).

2. Carefully measure the ingredients into the pan, except the bacon and onion.
3. Place all of the ingredients into a bucket in the right order, following the manual for your bread machine.
4. Close the cover.
5. Select the program of your bread machine to BASIC and choose the crust colour to MEDIUM.
6. Press START.
7. After the machine beeps, add the onion and bacon.
8. Wait until the program completes.
9. When done, take the bucket out and let it cool for 5-10 minutes.
10. Shake the loaf from the pan and let cool for 30 minutes on a cooling rack.
11. Slice, serve and enjoy the taste of fragrant Homemade Bread.
Nutrition Info: Calories: 391 Cal;Fat: 9.7 g;Cholesterol: 38 g;Sodium: 960 mg;Carbohydrates: 59.9 g;Total Sugars 1.2g;Protein 3.4g;Potassium 43mg

Classic Italian Herb Bread

Servings: 10
Cooking Time: 2 Hours
Ingredients:

- Active dry yeast – ¼ oz.
- Dried Italian seasoning – 4 tsps.
- Sugar – 3 tbsps.
- All-purpose flour – 4 cups
- Olive oil – 1/3 cup
- Water – 1 1/3 cups
- Salt – 2 tsps.

Directions:
1. Add olive oil and water to the bread pan. Add remaining ingredients except for yeast to the bread pan. Make a small hole in the flour with your finger and add yeast to the hole. Make sure yeast will not be mixed with any liquids. Select basic setting then select light/medium crust and start. Once loaf is done, remove the loaf pan from the machine. Allow it to cool for 10 minutes. Slice and serve.

Nutritious 9-grain Bread

Servings: 10
Cooking Time: 2 Hours
Ingredients:
- Warm water – ¾ cup+2 tbsps.
- Whole wheat flour – 1 cup.
- Bread flour – 1 cup.
- 9-grain cereal – ½ cup., crushed
- Salt – 1 tsp.
- Butter – 1 tbsp.
- Sugar – 2 tbsps.
- Milk powder – 1 tbsp.
- Active dry yeast – 2 tsps.

Directions:
1. Add all ingredients into the bread machine pan. Select whole wheat setting then select light/medium crust and start. Once loaf is done, remove the loaf pan from the machine. Allow it to cool for 10 minutes. Slice and serve.

Rosemary Cranberry Pecan Bread

Servings: 14 Slices
Cooking Time: 3 H.
Ingredients:
- 1⅓ cups water, plus
- 2 Tbsp water
- 2 Tbsp butter
- 2 tsp salt
- 4 cups bread flour
- ¾ cup dried sweetened cranberries
- ¾ cup toasted chopped pecans
- 2 Tbsp non-fat powdered milk
- ¼ cup sugar
- 2 tsp yeast

Directions:
1. Add each ingredient to the bread machine in the order and at the temperature recommended by your bread machine manufacturer.
2. Close the lid, select the basic bread, medium crust setting on your bread machine and press start.
3. When the bread machine has finished baking, remove the bread and put it on a cooling rack.

Lavender Buttermilk Bread

Servings: 14 Slices
Cooking Time: 3 H.
Ingredients:
- ½ cup water
- ⅞ cup buttermilk
- ¼ cup olive oil
- 3 Tbsp finely chopped fresh lavender leaves
- 1 ¼ tsp finely chopped fresh lavender flowers
- Grated zest of 1 lemon
- 4 cups bread flour
- 2 tsp salt
- 2 ¾ tsp bread machine yeast

Directions:
1. Add each ingredient to the bread machine in the order and at the temperature recommended by your bread machine manufacturer.
2. Close the lid, select the basic bread, medium crust setting on your bread machine and press start.
3. When the bread machine has finished baking, remove the bread and put it on a cooling rack.

Fragrant Cardamom Bread

Servings: 1 Loaf
Cooking Time: 10 Minutes
Ingredients:
- 12 slices bread (1½ pounds)
- ¾ cup milk, at 80°F to 90°F
- 1 egg, at room temperature
- 1½ teaspoons melted butter, cooled
- 3 tablespoons honey
- 1 teaspoon salt
- 1 teaspoon ground cardamom
- 3 cups white bread flour
- 1¼ teaspoons bread machine or instant yeast

Directions:
1. Preparing the Ingredients.
2. Choose the size of loaf of your preference and then measure the ingredients.
3. Add all of the ingredients mentioned previously in the list.
4. Close the lid after placing the pan in the bread machine.
5. Select the Bake cycle

6. Turn on the bread machine. Select the White/Basic setting, select the loaf size, and the crust color. Press start.

7. When the cycle is finished, carefully remove the pan from the bread maker and let it rest.

8. Remove the bread from the pan, put in a wire rack to Cool about 10 minutes. Slice

Herb And Garlic Cream Cheese Bread

Servings: 1 Loaf
Cooking Time: 10 Minutes
Ingredients:
- 12 slices bread (1½ pounds)
- ½ cup water, at 80°F to 90°F
- ½ cup herb and garlic cream cheese, at room temperature
- 1 egg, at room temperature
- 2 tablespoons melted butter, cooled
- 3 tablespoons sugar
- 1 teaspoon salt
- 3 cups white bread flour
- 1½ teaspoons bread machine or instant yeast

Directions:
1. Preparing the Ingredients.
2. Choose the size of loaf of your preference and then measure the ingredients.
3. Add all of the ingredients mentioned previously in the list.
4. Close the lid after placing the pan in the bread machine.
5. Select the Bake cycle
6. Turn on the bread machine. Select the White/Basic setting, select the loaf size, and the crust color. Press start.
7. When the cycle is finished, carefully remove the pan from the bread maker and let it rest.
8. Remove the bread from the pan, put in a wire rack to Cool about 10 minutes. Slice

Cornmeal Whole Wheat Bread

Servings: 10
Cooking Time: 2 Hours
Ingredients:
- Active dry yeast – 2 ½ tsps.
- Water – 1 1/3 cups.

- Sugar – 2 tbsps.
- Egg – 1, lightly beaten
- Butter – 2 tbsps.
- Salt – 1 ½ tsps.
- Cornmeal – ¾ cup.
- Whole wheat flour – ¾ cup.
- Bread flour – 2 ¾ cups.

Directions:
1. Add all ingredients to the bread machine pan according to the bread machine manufacturer instructions. Select basic bread setting then select medium crust and start. Once loaf is done, remove the loaf pan from the machine. Allow it to cool for 10 minutes. Slice and serve.

Garlic, Herb, And Cheese Bread

Servings: One Loaf (12 Slices)
Cooking Time: 15 Minutes
Ingredients:
- 1/2 cup ghee
- Six eggs
- 2 cups almond flour
- 1 tbsp baking powder
- 1/2 tsp xanthan gum
- 1 cup cheddar cheese, shredded
- 1 tbsp garlic powder
- 1 tbsp parsley
- 1/2 tbsp oregano
- 1/2 tsp salt

Directions:
1. Lightly beat eggs and ghee before pouring into bread machine pan.
2. Add the remaining ingredients to the pan.
3. Set bread machine to gluten-free.
4. When the bread is finished, remove the bread pan from the bread machine.
5. Let it cool for a while before transferring into a cooling rack.
6. You can store your bread for up to 5 days in the refrigerator.

Nutrition Info: Calories: 156 ;Carbohydrates: 4g;Protein: 5g;Fat: 13g

Healthy Spelt Bread

Servings: 10

Cooking Time: 40 Minutes

Ingredients:
- Milk – 1 ¼ cups.
- Sugar – 2 tbsps.
- Olive oil – 2 tbsps.
- Salt – 1 tsp.
- Spelt flour – 4 cups.
- Yeast – 2 ½ tsps.

Directions:
1. Add all ingredients to the bread machine pan according to the bread machine manufacturer instructions. Select basic bread setting then select light/medium crust and start. Once loaf is done, remove the loaf pan from the machine. Allow it to cool for 10 minutes. Slice and serve.

Whole Wheat Raisin Bread

Servings: 10
Cooking Time: 2 Hours

Ingredients:
- Whole wheat flour – 3 ½ cups
- Dry yeast – 2 tsps.
- Eggs – 2, lightly beaten
- Butter – ¼ cup, softened
- Water – ¾ cup
- Milk – 1/3 cup
- Salt – 1 tsp.
- Sugar – 1/3 cup
- Cinnamon – 4 tsps.
- Raisins – 1 cup

Directions:
1. Add water, milk, butter, and eggs to the bread pan. Add remaining ingredients except for yeast to the bread pan. Make a small hole into the flour with your finger and add yeast to the hole. Make sure yeast will not be mixed with any liquids. Select whole wheat setting then select light/medium crust and start. Once loaf is done, remove the loaf pan from the machine. Allow it to cool for 10 minutes. Slice and serve.

Spiced Raisin Bread

Servings: 24
Cooking Time: 3 Hours And 25 Minutes

Ingredients:

- Water – 1 cup, plus 2 tbsp.
- Raisins – ¾ cup
- Butter – 2 tbsp., softened
- Brown sugar – 2 tbsp.
- Ground cinnamon – 2 tsp.
- Salt – 1 tsp.
- Ground nutmeg – ¼ tsp.
- Ground cloves – ¼ tsp.
- Orange zest – ¼ tsp., grated
- Bread flour – 3 cups
- Active dry yeast – 2 ¼ tsp.

Directions:
1. Put all ingredients in the bread machine pan according to its order.
2. Select Basic cycle and choose crust. Press Start.
3. When the bread is done, remove it.
4. Cool, slice, and serve.

Nutrition Info: (Per Serving): Calories: 78; Total Fat: 1 g; Saturated Fat: 1 g; Carbohydrates: 4 g; Cholesterol: 3 mg; Fiber: 1 g; Calcium: 7 mg; Sodium: 106 mg; Protein: 2 g

Pesto Nut Bread

Servings: 14 Slices
Cooking Time: 10 Minutes

Ingredients:
- 1 cup plus 2 Tbsp water
- 3 cups Gold Medal Better for Bread flour
- 2 Tbsp sugar
- 1 tsp salt
- 1¼ tsp bread machine or quick active dry yeast
- For the pesto filling:
- ⅓ cup basil pesto
- 2 Tbsp Gold Medal Better for Bread flour
- ⅓ cup pine nuts

Directions:
1. Preparing the Ingredients
2. Add each ingredient to the bread machine in the order and at the temperature recommended by your bread machine manufacturer.
3. Select the Bake cycle
4. Close the lid, select the basic bread, medium crust setting on your bread machine, and press start.

5. In a small bowl, combine pesto and 2 Tbsp of flour until well blended. Stir in the pine nuts. Add the filling 5 minutes before the last kneading cycle ends.

6. When the bread machine has finished baking, remove the bread and put it on a cooling rack.

Honeyed Bulgur Bread

Servings: 1 Loaf
Cooking Time: 10 Minutes
Ingredients:

- 12 slice bread (1½ pounds)
- ¾ cup boiling water
- 3 tablespoons bulgur wheat
- 3 tablespoons quick oats
- 2 eggs, at room temperature
- 1½ tablespoons melted butter, cooled
- 2¼ tablespoons honey
- 1 teaspoon salt
- 2¼ cups white bread flour
- 1½ teaspoons bread machine or instant yeast

Directions:

1. Preparing the Ingredients.
2. Place the water, bulgur, and oats in the bucket of your bread machine for 30 minutes or until the liquid is 80°F to 90°F.
3. Place the remaining ingredients in your bread machine as recommended by the manufacturer.
4. Select the Bake cycle
5. Turn on the bread machine. Select the White/Basic setting, select the loaf size, and the crust color. Press start.
6. When the cycle is finished, carefully remove the pan from the bread maker and let it rest.
7. Remove the bread from the pan, put in a wire rack to Cool about 5 minutes. Slice

Cinnamon Bread

Servings: 1 Loaf
Cooking Time: 10 Minutes
Ingredients:

- 12 slices bread (1½ pounds)
- 1 cup milk, at 80°F to 90°F
- 1 egg, at room temperature
- ¼ cup melted butter, cooled
- ½ cup sugar

- ½ teaspoon salt
- 1½ teaspoons ground cinnamon
- 3 cups white bread flour
- 2 teaspoons bread machine or active dry yeast

Directions:

1. Preparing the Ingredients.
2. Choose the size of loaf of your preference and then measure the ingredients.
3. Add all of the ingredients mentioned previously in the list.
4. Close the lid after placing the pan in the bread machine.
5. Select the Bake cycle
6. Turn on the bread machine. Select the White/Basic setting, select the loaf size, and the crust color. Press start.
7. When the cycle is finished, carefully remove the pan from the bread maker and let it rest.
8. Remove the bread from the pan, put in a wire rack to Cool about 10 minutes. Slice

Grain, Seed And Nut Bread

Servings: 1 Loaf
Cooking Time: 10 Minutes
Ingredients:

- ¼ cup water
- 1 egg
- 3 Tbsp honey
- 1½ tsp butter, softened
- 3¼ cups bread flour
- 1 cup milk
- 1 tsp salt
- ¼ tsp baking soda
- 1 tsp ground cinnamon
- 2½ tsp active dry yeast
- ¾ cup dried cranberries
- ½ cup chopped walnuts
- 1 Tbsp white vinegar
- ½ tsp sugar

Directions:

1. Preparing the Ingredients.
2. Choose the size of loaf of your preference and then measure the ingredients.
3. Add all of the ingredients mentioned previously in the list.

4. Close the lid after placing the pan in the bread machine.

5. Select the Bake cycle

6. Turn on the bread machine. Select the White/Basic setting, select the loaf size, and the crust color. Press start.

7. When the cycle is finished, carefully remove the pan from the bread maker and let it rest.

8. Remove the bread from the pan, put in a wire rack to Cool about 10 minutes. Slice

Caraway Rye Bread

Servings: 1 Loaf
Cooking Time: 10 Minutes
Ingredients:
- 12 slice bread (1½ pounds)
- 1⅛ cups water, at 80°F to 90°F
- 1¾ tablespoons melted butter, cooled
- 3 tablespoons dark brown sugar
- 1½ tablespoons dark molasses
- 1⅛ teaspoons salt
- 1½ teaspoons caraway seed
- ¾ cup dark rye flour
- 2 cups white bread flour
- 1⅛ teaspoons bread machine or instant yeast

Directions:
1. Preparing the Ingredients.
2. Choose the size of loaf of your preference and then measure the ingredients.
3. Add all of the ingredients mentioned previously in the list.
4. Close the lid after placing the pan in the bread machine.
5. Select the Bake cycle
6. Turn on the bread machine. Select the White/Basic setting, select the loaf size, and the crust color. Press start.
7. When the cycle is finished, carefully remove the pan from the bread maker and let it rest.
8. Remove the bread from the pan, put in a wire rack to Cool about 10 minutes. Slice

Aromatic Lavender Bread

Servings: 1 Loaf
Cooking Time: 10 Minutes
Ingredients:

- 16 slices bread (2 pounds)
- 1½ cups milk, at 80°F to 90°F
- 2 tablespoons melted butter, cooled
- 2 tablespoons sugar
- 2 teaspoons salt
- 2 teaspoons chopped fresh lavender flowers
- 1 teaspoon lemon zest
- ½ teaspoon chopped fresh thyme
- 4 cups white bread flour
- 1½ teaspoons bread machine or instant yeast

Directions:
1. Preparing the Ingredients.
2. Choose the size of loaf of your preference and then measure the ingredients.
3. Add all of the ingredients mentioned previously in the list.
4. Close the lid after placing the pan in the bread machine.
5. Select the Bake cycle
6. Turn on the bread machine. Select the White/Basic setting, select the loaf size, and the crust color. Press start.
7. When the cycle is finished, carefully remove the pan from the bread maker and let it rest.
8. Remove the bread from the pan, put in a wire rack to Cool about 10 minutes. Slice

Hazelnut Honey Bread

Servings: 1 Loaf
Cooking Time: 10 Minutes
Ingredients:
- 16 slices bread (2 pounds)
- 1⅓ cups lukewarm milk
- 2 eggs, at room temperature
- 5 tablespoons unsalted butter, melted
- ¼ cup honey
- 1 teaspoon pure vanilla extract
- 1 teaspoon table salt
- 4 cups white bread flour
- 1 cup toasted hazelnuts, finely ground
- 2 teaspoons bread machine yeast

Directions:
1. Preparing the Ingredients.
2. Choose the size of loaf of your preference and then measure the ingredients.
3. Add all of the ingredients mentioned previously in the list.

4. Close the lid after placing the pan in the bread machine.
5. Select the Bake cycle
6. Turn on the bread machine. Select the White/Basic setting, select the loaf size, and the crust color. Press start.
7. When the cycle is finished, carefully remove the pan from the bread maker and let it rest.
8. Remove the bread from the pan, put in a wire rack to Cool about 10 minutes. Slice

Cardamom Cranberry Bread

Servings: 14 Slices
Cooking Time: 3 H.
Ingredients:
- 1¾ cups water
- 2 Tbsp brown sugar
- 1½ tsp salt
- 2 Tbsp coconut oil
- 4 cups flour
- 2 tsp cinnamon
- 2 tsp cardamom
- 1 cup dried cranberries
- 2 tsp yeast

Directions:
1. Add each ingredient except the dried cranberries to the bread machine in the order and at the temperature recommended by your bread machine manufacturer.
2. Close the lid, select the basic bread, medium crust setting on your bread machine and press start.
3. Add the dried cranberries 5 to 10 minutes before the last kneading cycle ends.
4. When the bread machine has finished baking, remove the bread and put it on a cooling rack.

Molasses Candied-ginger Bread

Servings: 1 Loaf
Cooking Time: 10 Minutes
Ingredients:
- 12 slices bread (1½ pounds)
- 1 cup milk, at 80°F to 90°F
- 1 egg, at room temperature
- ¼ cup dark molasses
- 3 tablespoons butter, melted and cooled
- ½ teaspoon salt
- ¼ cup chopped candied ginger

- ½ cup quick oats
- 3 cups white bread flour
- 2 teaspoons bread machine or instant yeast

Directions:
1. Preparing the Ingredients.
2. Choose the size of loaf of your preference and then measure the ingredients.
3. Add all of the ingredients mentioned previously in the list.
4. Close the lid after placing the pan in the bread machine.
5. Select the Bake cycle
6. Turn on the bread machine. Select the White/Basic setting, select the loaf size, and the crust color. Press start.
7. When the cycle is finished, carefully remove the pan from the bread maker and let it rest.
8. Remove the bread from the pan, put in a wire rack to Cool about 5 minutes. Slice

Oatmeal Sunflower Bread

Servings: 10
Cooking Time: 3 Hours 30 Minutes
Ingredients:
- Water – 1 cup.
- Honey – ¼ cup.
- Butter – 2 tbsps., softened
- Bread flour – 3 cups.
- Old fashioned oats – ½ cup.
- Milk powder – 2 tbsps.
- Salt – 1 ¼ tsps.
- Active dry yeast – 2 ¼ tsps.
- Sunflower seeds – ½ cup.

Directions:
1. Add all ingredients except for sunflower seeds into the bread machine pan. Select basic setting then select light/medium crust and press start. Add sunflower seeds just before the final kneading cycle. Once loaf is done, remove the loaf pan from the machine. Allow it to cool for 10 minutes. Slice and serve.

Tuscan Herb Bread

Servings: 10
Cooking Time: 2 Hours
Ingredients:
- Yeast – 2 tsps.

- Bread flour – 2 1/2 cups
- Italian seasoning – 2 tbsps.
- Sugar – 2 tbsps.
- Olive oil – 2 tbsps.
- Warm water – 1 cup
- Salt – 1 tsp.

Directions:

1. Add olive oil and water to the bread pan. Add remaining ingredients except for yeast to the bread pan. Make a small hole into the flour with your finger and add yeast to the hole. Make sure yeast will not be mixed with any liquids. Select basic setting then select light/medium crust and start. Once loaf is done, remove the loaf pan from the machine. Allow it to cool for 10 minutes. Slice and serve.

Whole-wheat Seed Bread

Servings: 1 Loaf
Cooking Time: 10 Minutes
Ingredients:

- 12 slice bread (1½ pounds)
- 1⅛ cups water, at 80°F to 90°F
- 1½ tablespoons honey
- 1½ tablespoons melted butter, cooled
- ¾ teaspoon salt
- 2½ cups whole-wheat flour
- ¾ cup white bread flour
- 3 tablespoons raw sunflower seeds
- 1 tablespoon sesame seeds
- 1½ teaspoons bread machine or instant yeast

Directions:

1. Preparing the Ingredients.
2. Choose the size of loaf of your preference and then measure the ingredients.
3. Add all of the ingredients mentioned previously in the list.
4. Close the lid after placing the pan in the bread machine.
5. Select the Bake cycle
6. Turn on the bread machine. Select the Whole-Wheat/Whole-Grain bread, select the loaf size, and select light or medium crust. Press start.
7. When the cycle is finished, carefully remove the pan from the bread maker and let it rest.
8. Remove the bread from the pan, put in a wire rack to Cool about 5 minutes. Slice

Simple Garlic Bread

Servings: 1 Loaf
Cooking Time: 10 Minutes
Ingredients:

- 12 slices bread (1½ pounds)
- 1 cup milk, at 70°F to 80°F
- 1½ tablespoons melted butter, cooled
- 1 tablespoon sugar
- 1½ teaspoons salt
- 2 teaspoons garlic powder
- 2 teaspoons chopped fresh parsley
- 3 cups white bread flour
- 1¾ teaspoons bread machine or instant yeast

Directions:

1. Preparing the Ingredients.
2. Choose the size of loaf of your preference and then measure the ingredients.
3. Add all of the ingredients mentioned previously in the list.
4. Close the lid after placing the pan in the bread machine.
5. Select the Bake cycle
6. Turn on the bread machine. Select the White/Basic setting, select the loaf size, and the crust color. Press start.
7. When the cycle is finished, carefully remove the pan from the bread maker and let it rest.
8. Remove the bread from the pan, put in a wire rack to Cool about 10 minutes. Slice

Honey-spice Egg Bread

Servings: 1 Loaf
Cooking Time: 10 Minutes
Ingredients:

- 12 slices bread (1½ pounds)
- 1 cup milk, at 80°F to 90°F
- 2 eggs, at room temperature
- 1½ tablespoons melted butter, cooled
- 2 tablespoons honey
- 1 teaspoon salt
- 1 teaspoon ground cinnamon
- ½ teaspoon ground cardamom
- ½ teaspoon ground nutmeg
- 3 cups white bread flour
- 2 teaspoons bread machine or instant yeast

Directions:

1. Preparing the Ingredients.

2. Choose the size of loaf of your preference and then measure the ingredients.
3. Add all of the ingredients mentioned previously in the list.
4. Close the lid after placing the pan in the bread machine.
5. Select the Bake cycle
6. Turn on the bread machine. Select the White/Basic setting, select the loaf size, and the crust color. Press start.
7. When the cycle is finished, carefully remove the pan from the bread maker and let it rest.
8. Remove the bread from the pan, put in a wire rack to Cool about 10 minutes. Slice

Cajun Bread

Servings: 14 Slices
Cooking Time: 10 Minutes
Ingredients:
- ½ cup water
- ¼ cup chopped onion
- ¼ cup chopped green bell pepper
- 2 tsp finely chopped garlic
- 2 tsp soft butter
- 2 cups bread flour
- 1 Tbsp sugar
- 1 tsp Cajun
- ½ tsp salt
- 1 tsp active dry yeast

Directions:
1. Preparing the Ingredients
2. Add each ingredient to the bread machine in the order and at the temperature recommended by your bread machine manufacturer.

3. Select the Bake cycle
4. Close the lid, select the basic bread, medium crust setting on your bread machine and press start.
5. When the bread machine has finished baking, remove the bread and put it on a cooling rack.

Olive Bread

Servings: 14 Slices
Cooking Time: 3 H.
Ingredients:
- ½ cup brine from olive jar
- Add warm water (110°F) To make 1½ cup when combined with brine
- 2 Tbsp olive oil
- 3 cups bread flour
- 1⅔ cups whole wheat flour
- 1½ tsp salt
- 2 Tbsp sugar
- 1½ tsp dried leaf basil
- 2 tsp active dry yeast
- ⅔ cup finely chopped Kalamata olives

Directions:
1. Add each ingredient except the olives to the bread machine in the order and at the temperature recommended by your bread machine manufacturer.
2. Close the lid, select the wheat, medium crust setting on your bread machine and press start.
3. Add the olives 10 minutes before the last kneading cycle ends.
4. When the bread machine has finished baking, remove the bread and put it on a cooling rack.

CHEESE & SWEET BREAD

Sugared Doughnuts

Servings: 20 Doughnuts
Cooking Time: 30 Minutes Plus Fermenting Time

Ingredients:

- 2/3 cup milk
- ¼ cup water
- ¼ cup butter, softened
- 1 egg
- 3 cups bread flour
- ¼ cup sugar
- 1 teaspoon salt
- 2½ teaspoons bread machine or fast-acting dry yeast
- Vegetable oil
- Additional sugar, if desired

Directions:

1. Preparing the Ingredients.
2. Choose the size of loaf of your preference and then measure the ingredients.
3. Add all of the ingredients mentioned previously in the list, except for the vegetable oil and additional sugar. Close the lid after placing the pan in the bread machine.
4. Select the Bake cycle
5. Select Dough/Manual cycle. Do not use delay cycle. Remove dough from pan, using lightly floured hands. Cover and let rest 10 minutes on lightly floured board. Roll dough to 3/8-inch thickness on lightly floured board. Cut with floured doughnut cutter. Cover and let rise on board 35 to 45 minutes or until slightly raised.
6. In deep fryer or heavy Dutch oven, heat 2 to 3 inches oil to 375°F. Fry doughnuts in oil, 2 or 3 at a time, turning as they rise to the surface. Fry 2 to 3 minutes or until golden brown on both sides. Remove from oil with slotted spoon to cooling rack. Roll warm doughnuts in sugar.

Beer And Pretzel Bread

Servings: 12 Slices
Cooking Time: 10 Minutes Plus Fermenting Time

Ingredients:

- ¾ cup regular or nonalcoholic beer
- 1/3 cup water
- 2 tablespoons butter, softened
- 3 cups bread flour
- 1 tablespoon packed brown sugar
- 1 teaspoon ground mustard
- 1 teaspoon salt
- 1½ teaspoons bread machine yeast
- ½ cup bite-size pretzel pieces, about 1×¾ inch, or pretzel rods, cut into 1-inch pieces

Directions:

1. Preparing the Ingredients.
2. Measure carefully, placing all ingredients except pretzels in bread machine pan in order recommended by the manufacturer.
3. Select the Bake cycle
4. Select Basic/White cycle. Use Medium or Light crust color. Do not use delay cycle.
5. Add pretzels 5 minutes before the last kneading cycle ends. Remove baked bread from pan; cool on cooling rack.

Everyday Fruit Bread

Servings: 15
Cooking Time: 3 Hours And 25 Minutes

Ingredients:

- Egg – 1
- Water – 1 cup, plus 2 tbsp.
- Ground cardamom – ½ tsp.
- Salt – 1 tsp.
- Sugar – 1 ½ tbsp.
- Butter – ¼ cup
- Bread flour – 3 cups
- Bread machine yeast – 1 tsp.
- Raisins – 1/3 cup
- Mixed candied fruit – 1/3 cup

Directions:

1. Place all ingredients (except fruit and raisins) in the bread machine according to machine recommendation.
2. Select Basic White or Fruit and Nut setting.
3. Add the fruit and raisins after the beep.
4. When finished, remove the bread.
5. Cool, slice, and serve.

Nutrition Info: (Per Serving): Calories: 144; Total Fat: 3.6 g; Saturated Fat: 2.1 g; Carbohydrates: 24.6 g;

Cholesterol: 19 mg; Fiber: 1 g; Calcium: 9 mg; Sodium: 183 mg; Protein: 3.2 g

Nutrition Info: (Per Serving):Calories 156, fat 3.7 g, carbs 26.3 g, sodium 248 mg, protein 4.3 g

Cinnamon Rum Bread

Servings: 1 Loaf

Ingredients:

- 16 slice bread (2 pounds)
- 1⅛ cups lukewarm water
- 1 egg, at room temperature
- ¼ cup butter, melted and cooled
- ¼ cup sugar
- 4 teaspoons rum extract
- 1⅔ teaspoons table salt
- 4 cups white bread flour
- 1⅓ teaspoons ground cinnamon
- ¼ teaspoon ground nutmeg
- 1⅓ teaspoons bread machine yeast
- 12 slice bread (1½ pounds)
- ¾ cup lukewarm water
- 1 egg, at room temperature
- 3 tablespoons butter, melted and cooled
- 3 tablespoons sugar
- 1 tablespoon rum extract
- 1¼ teaspoons table salt
- 3 cups white bread flour
- 1 teaspoon ground cinnamon
- ¼ teaspoon ground nutmeg
- 1 teaspoon bread machine yeast

Directions:

1. Choose the size of loaf you would like to make and measure your ingredients.
2. Add the ingredients to the bread pan in the order listed above.
3. Place the pan in the bread machine and close the lid.
4. Turn on the bread maker. Select the Sweet setting, then the loaf size, and finally the crust color. Start the cycle.
5. When the cycle is finished and the bread is baked, carefully remove the pan from the machine. Use a potholder as the handle will be very hot. Let rest for a few minutes.
6. Remove the bread from the pan and allow to cool on a wire rack for at least 10 minutes before slicing.

Cheese Pepperoni Bread

Servings: 10
Cooking Time: 2 Hours

Ingredients:

- Pepperoni – 2/3 cup, diced
- Active dry yeast – 1 ½ tsps.
- Bread flour – 3 ¼ cups.
- Dried oregano – 1 ½ tsps.
- Garlic salt – 1 ½ tsps.
- Sugar – 2 tbsps.
- Mozzarella cheese – 1/3 cup., shredded
- Warm water – 1 cup+2 tbsps.

Directions:

1. Add all ingredients except for pepperoni into the bread machine pan. Select basic setting then select medium crust and press start. Add pepperoni just before the final kneading cycle. Once loaf is done, remove the loaf pan from the machine. Allow it to cool for 10 minutes. Slice and serve.

Dry Fruit Bread

Servings: 12
Cooking Time: 3 Hours And 25 Minutes

Ingredients:

- Water – 1 cup, plus 2 tbsp.
- Egg – 1
- Butter – 3 tbsp., softened
- Packed brown sugar – ¼ cup
- Salt – 1 ½ tsp.
- Ground nutmeg – ¼ tsp.
- Dash allspice
- Bread flour – 3 ¾ cups, plus 1 tbsp.
- Active dry yeast – 2 tsp.
- Dried fruit – 1 cup
- Chopped pecans – 1/3 cup

Directions:

1. Add everything (except fruit and pecans) in the bread machine according to the machine recommendations.
2. Select Basic bread cycle.
3. Add fruit and pecans at the beep.
4. Remove the bread when done.

5. Cool, slice, and serve.

Nutrition Info: (Per Serving): Calories: 214; Total Fat: 6 g; Saturated Fat: 2 g; Carbohydrates: 36 g; Cholesterol: 25 mg; Fiber: 2 g; Calcium: 38 mg; Sodium: 330 mg; Protein: 6 g

Cinnamon Bread

Servings: 1 Loaf
Cooking Time: 10 Minutes Plus Fermenting Time
Ingredients:
- 12 slice bread (1½ pounds)
- ¾ cup lukewarm water
- 1 egg, at room temperature
- 3 tablespoons butter, melted and cooled
- 3 tablespoons sugar
- 1 tablespoon rum extract
- 1¼ teaspoons table salt
- 3 cups white bread flour
- 1 teaspoon ground cinnamon
- ¼ teaspoon ground nutmeg
- 1 teaspoon bread machine yeast

Directions:
1. Preparing the Ingredients.
2. Choose the size of loaf of your preference and then measure the ingredients.
3. Add all of the ingredients mentioned previously in the list.
4. Close the lid after placing the pan in the bread machine.
5. Select the Bake cycle
6. Turn on the bread machine. Select the Basic/White setting, select the loaf size, and the crust color. Press start.
7. When the cycle is finished, carefully remove the pan from the bread maker and let it rest.
8. Remove the bread from the pan, put in a wire rack to Cool about 5 minutes. Slice

Hawaiian Sweet Bread

Servings: 1 Loaf
Cooking Time: 2 Hour
Ingredients:
- 3/4 cup pineapple juice
- One egg
- Two tablespoons vegetable oil
- 2 1/2 tablespoons honey
- 3/4 teaspoon salt
- 3 cups bread flour
- Two tablespoons dry milk
- Two teaspoons fast-rising yeast

Directions:
1. Place ingredients in bread machine container.
2. Select the white bread cycle.
3. Press the start button.
4. Take out the pan when done and set aside for 10 minutes.

Nutrition Info: Calories 169;Carbohydrates: 25g;Total Fat 5g;Cholesterol 25mg;Protein 4g;Fiber 1g;Sugar 5g;Sodium 165mg;Potassium 76mg

Walnut Cocoa Bread

Servings: 14 Servings
Cooking Time: 20 Minutes Plus Fermenting Time
Ingredients:
- ⅔ cup milk
- ⅓ cup water
- 5 Tbsp butter, softened
- ⅓ cup packed brown sugar
- 5 Tbsp baking cocoa
- 1 tsp salt
- 3 cups bread flour
- 2¼ tsp active dry yeast
- ⅔ cup chopped walnuts, toasted

Directions:
1. Preparing the Ingredients
2. Add each ingredient except the walnuts to the bread machine in the order and at the temperature recommended by your bread machine manufacturer.
3. Select the Bake cycle
4. Close the lid, select the sweet loaf, low crust setting on your bread machine, and press start.
5. Just before the final kneading, add the walnuts.
6. When the bread machine has finished baking, remove the bread and put it on a cooling rack.

Zesty Cheddar Bread

Servings: 1 Loaf
Cooking Time: 10 Minutes
Ingredients:
- 12 slice bread (1½ pounds)

- 1 cup buttermilk
- 1/3 cup butter, melted
- 1 tablespoon sugar
- 2 tablespoons finely chopped chipotle chiles in adobo sauce (from 7-oz can) 2 eggs
- 2 cups all-purpose flour
- 1 cup shredded Cheddar cheese (4 oz)
- 2 teaspoons baking powder
- 1 teaspoon baking soda
- ½ teaspoon salt

Directions:
1. Preparing the Ingredients.
2. Choose the size of loaf of your preference and then measure the ingredients.
3. Add all of the ingredients mentioned previously in the list.
4. Close the lid after placing the pan in the bread machine.
5. Select the Bake cycle
6. Turn on the bread machine. Select the White/Basic setting, select the loaf size, and the crust color. Press start.
7. When the cycle is finished, carefully remove the pan from the bread maker and let it rest.
8. Remove the bread from the pan, put in a wire rack to Cool about 5 minutes. Serve warm

Parmesan Cheese Bread

Servings: 8
Cooking Time: 3 Hours And 25 Minutes
Ingredients:
- Wheat bread flour - 2½ cups
- Fresh bread machine yeast - 1½ tsp.
- Whole milk - ½ cup, lukewarm
- Butter - 1 tbsp., melted
- Sugar - 2 tbsp.
- Kosher salt - ½ tsp.
- Whole eggs – 2
- Fresh/dried rosemary -2 tsp., ground
- Parmesan - 3 tbsp. (divided - 2 tbsp. for dough and 1 tbsp. for sprinkling)
- Garlic - 2 cloves, crushed

Directions:
1. Place all the dry and liquid ingredients (except for parmesan, yeast, milk, rosemary, and garlic) in

the bread pan according to bread machine recommendations.
2. Dissolve the yeast in the warm milk and add.
3. Add the garlic, parmesan, and rosemary after the beep.
4. Choose Basic cycle and Light crust.
5. Remove the bread when done.
6. Cool, slice, and serve.
Nutrition Info: (Per Serving): Calories: 212; Total Fat: 4.6 g; Saturated Fat: 2.1 g; Carbohydrates: 34.8 g; Cholesterol: 49 mg; Fiber: 1.5 g; Calcium: 18 mg; Sodium: 214 mg; Protein: 7.6 g

Almond Chocolate Chip Bread

Servings: 14 Slices
Cooking Time: 10 Minutes Plus Fermenting Time
Ingredients:
- 1 cup plus 2 Tbsp water
- 2 Tbsp softened butter
- ½ tsp vanilla
- 3 cups Gold Medal Better for Bread flour
- ¾ cup semisweet chocolate chips
- 3 Tbsp sugar
- 1 Tbsp dry milk
- ¾ tsp salt
- 1½ tsp quick active dry yeast
- ⅓ cup sliced almonds

Directions:
1. Preparing the Ingredients
2. Add each ingredient except the almonds to the bread machine in the order and at the temperature recommended by your bread machine manufacturer.
3. Select the Bake cycle
4. Close the lid, select the sweet loaf, low crust setting on your bread machine, and press start.
5. Add almonds 10 minutes before last kneading cycle ends. When the bread machine has finished baking, remove the bread and put it on a cooling rack.

Prosciutto Parmesan Breadsticks

Servings: 12
Cooking Time: 10 Minutes
Ingredients:
- 1 1/3 cups warm water
- 1 tablespoon butter

- 1 1/2 tablespoons sugar
- 1 1/2 teaspoons salt
- 4 cups bread flour
- 2 teaspoons yeast
- For the topping:
- 1/2 pound prosciutto, sliced very thin
- 1/2 cup of grated parmesan cheese
- 1 egg yolk
- 1 tablespoon of water

Directions:
1. Preparing the Ingredients
2. Place the first set of dough ingredients (except yeast) in the bread pan in the order indicated. Do not add any of the topping ingredients yet. Make a well in the center of the dry ingredients and add the yeast.
3. Select the Bake cycle
4. Select the Dough cycle on the bread machine. When finished, drop the dough onto a lightly-floured surface.
5. Roll the dough out flat to about 1/4-inch thick, or about half a centimeter. Cover with plastic wrap and let rise for 20 to 30 minutes.
6. Sprinkle dough evenly with parmesan and carefully lay the prosciutto slices on the surface of the dough to cover as much of it as possible. Preheat an oven to 400°F.
7. Cut the dough into 12 long strips, about one inch wide. Twist each end in opposite directions, twisting the toppings into the bread stick. Place the breadsticks onto a lightly greased baking sheet. Whisk the egg yolk and water together in a small mixing bowl and lightly baste each breadstick. Bake for 8 to 10 minutes or until golden brown.
8. Remove from oven and serve warm.

Caramel Apple And Pecan Bread

Servings: 1 Loaf
Cooking Time: 10 Minutes Plus Fermenting Time
Ingredients:
- 12 slice bread (1½ pounds)
- 1 cup water
- 2 tablespoons butter, softened
- 3 cups bread flour
- ¼ cup packed brown sugar
- ¾ teaspoon ground cinnamon
- 1 teaspoon salt
- 2 teaspoons bread machine or fast-acting dry yeast
- ½ cup chopped unpeeled apple
- 1/3 cup coarsely chopped pecans, toasted

Directions:
1. Preparing the Ingredients.
2. Choose the size of loaf of your preference and then measure the ingredients.
3. Add all of the ingredients mentioned previously in the list except apple and pecans in bread maker. Add apple and pecans at the Raisin/Nut signal or 5 to 10 minutes before last kneading cycle ends.
4. Select the Bake cycle
5. Program the machine for Basic/White bread and press Start.
6. When the cycle is finished, carefully remove the pan from the bread maker and let it rest.
7. Remove the bread from the pan, put in a wire rack to Cool about 5 minutes. Slice

Apricot–cream Cheese Ring

Servings: 10 Servings
Cooking Time: 10 Minutes
Ingredients:
- 1/3 cup water
- 2 tablespoons butter, softened
- 1 egg
- 2 cups bread flour
- 2 tablespoons sugar
- ½ teaspoon salt
- 1¾ teaspoons bread machine or fast-acting dry yeast
- filling
- 1 package (3 oz) cream cheese, softened
- 1½ tablespoons bread flour
- ¼ cup apricot preserves
- 1 egg, beaten
- 2 tablespoons sliced almonds

Directions:
1. Preparing the Ingredients.
2. Measure carefully, placing all bread dough ingredients in bread machine pan in the order recommended by the manufacturer.
3. Select Dough/Manual cycle. Do not use delay cycle.

4. Remove dough from pan, using lightly floured hands. Cover and let rest 10 minutes on lightly floured surface. In small bowl, mix cream cheese and 1½ tablespoons flour.

5. 4 Grease 9-inch round pan with shortening. Roll dough into 15-inch round.

6. Place in pan, letting side of dough hang over edge of pan. Spread cream cheese mixture over dough in pan; spoon apricot preserves onto cream cheese mixture.

7. Select the Bake cycle

8. Make cuts along edge of dough at 1-inch intervals to about ½ inch above cream cheese mixture. Twist pairs of dough strips and fold over cream cheese mixture.

9. Cover and let rise in warm place 40 to 50 minutes or until almost double.

10. 5 Heat oven to 375°F. Brush beaten egg over dough. Sprinkle with almonds.

11. Bake 30 to 35 minutes or until golden brown. Cool at least 30 minutes before cutting.

Apple Cider Bread

Servings: 1 Loaf

Cooking Time: 10 Minutes Plus Fermenting Time

Ingredients:
- 8 slices bread (1 pound)
- ¼ cup milk, at 80°F to 90°F
- 2 tablespoons apple cider, at room temperature
- 2 tablespoons sugar
- 4 teaspoons melted butter, cooled
- 1 tablespoon honey
- ¼ teaspoon salt
- 2 cups white bread flour
- ¾ teaspoons bread machine or instant yeast
- ⅔ apple, peeled, cored, and finely diced

Directions:
1. Preparing the Ingredients.
2. Place the ingredients, except the apple, in your bread machine as recommended by the manufacturer.
3. Select the Bake cycle
4. Program the machine for Basic/White bread, select light or medium crust, and press Start.
5. Add the apple when the machine signals or 5 minutes before the last kneading cycle is complete.

6. When the cycle is finished, carefully remove the pan from the bread maker and let it rest.

7. Remove the bread from the pan, put in a wire rack to Cool about 5 minutes. Slice

Easy Donuts

Servings: 12

Cooking Time: 1 Hour

Ingredients:
- 2/3 cups milk, room temperature
- 1/4 cup water, room temperature
- ½ cup of warm water
- 1/4 cup softened butter
- One egg slightly has beaten
- 1/4 cup granulated sugar
- 1 tsp salt
- 3 cups bread machine flour
- 2 1/2 tsp bread machine yeast
- oil for deep frying
- 1/4 cup confectioners' sugar

Directions:
1. Place the milk, water, butter, egg sugar, salt, flour, and yeast in a pan.
2. Select dough setting and push start. Press the start button.
3. When the process is complete, remove dough from the pan and transfer it to a lightly floured surface.
4. Using a rolling pin lightly dusted with flour, roll dough to ½ inch thickness.
5. Cut with a floured dusted donut cutter or circle cookie cutter.
6. Transfer donuts to a baking sheet that has been covered with wax paper. Place another layer of paper on top, then cover with a clean tea towel. Let rise 30-40 minutes.
7. Heat vegetable oil to 375º (190ºCº) in a deep-fryer or large, heavy pot.
8. Fry donuts 2-3 at a time until golden brown on both sides for about 3 minutes.
9. Drain on a paper towel.
10. Sprinkle with confectioners' sugar.

Nutrition Info: Calories 180;Carbohydrates: 30g;Total Fat 5g;Cholesterol 25mg;Protein 4g;Fiber 2g;Sugar 7g;Sodium 240mg;Potassium 64mg

Moist Cheddar Cheese Bread

Servings: 10
Cooking Time: 3 Hours 45 Minutes
Ingredients:
- Milk – 1 cup
- Butter – ½ cup, melted
- All-purpose flour – 3 cups
- Cheddar cheese – 2 cups, shredded
- Garlic powder – ½ tsp.
- Kosher salt – 2 tsps.
- Sugar – 1 tbsp.
- Active dry yeast – 1 ¼ oz.

Directions:
1. Add milk and butter into the bread pan. Add remaining ingredients except for yeast to the bread pan. Make a small hole into the flour with your finger and add yeast to the hole. Make sure yeast will not be mixed with any liquids. Select basic setting then select light crust and start. Once loaf is done, remove the loaf pan from the machine. Allow it to cool for 10 minutes. Slice and serve.

Cocoa Banana Bread

Servings: 1 Loaf
Cooking Time: 10 Minutes Plus Fermenting Time
Ingredients:
- 12 slice bread (1½ pounds)
- 3 bananas, mashed
- 2 eggs, at room temperature
- ¾ cup packed light brown sugar
- ½ cup unsalted butter, melted
- ½ cup sour cream, at room temperature
- ¼ cup sugar
- 1½ teaspoons pure vanilla extract
- 1 cup all-purpose flour
- ½ cup quick oats
- 2 tablespoons unsweetened cocoa powder
- 1 teaspoon baking soda

Directions:
1. Preparing the Ingredients.
2. Choose the size of loaf of your preference and then measure the ingredients.
3. Add all of the ingredients mentioned previously in the list.

4. Close the lid after placing the pan in the bread machine.
5. Select the Bake cycle
6. Turn on the bread machine. Select the Quick/Rapid setting, select the loaf size, and the crust color. Press start.
7. When the cycle is finished, carefully remove the pan from the bread maker and let it rest.
8. Remove the bread from the pan, put in a wire rack to Cool about 5 minutes. Slice

Peach Bread

Servings: 10
Cooking Time: 3 Hours And 48 Minutes
Ingredients:
- Wholemeal flour – 4 cups
- Bread machine yeast – 2 tsp.
- Lukewarm water – 1 ¼ cups
- Flaxseed oil – 1 ½ tsp.
- Brown sugar – 1 ½ tsp.
- Kosher salt – 1 ½ tsp.
- Peaches – 2, peeled and diced

Directions:
1. Add everything in the bread machine (except the peaches) according to bread machine recommendations.
2. Select Whole-Grain and Medium crust.
3. Add the peaches after the beep.
4. Remove the bread when done.
5. Cool, slice, and serve.

Nutrition Info: (Per Serving): Calories: 246; Total Fat: 4 g; Saturated Fat: 0.3 g; Carbohydrates: 44.3 g; Cholesterol: 0 mg; Fiber: 6.4 g; Calcium: 50 mg; Sodium: 440 mg; Protein: 8.2 g

Strawberry Bread

Servings: 10
Cooking Time: 3 Hours And 25 Minutes
Ingredients:
- Lukewarm water – 1 ¾ cups
- Kosher salt – 2 ½ tsp.
- Bread machine flour – 4 cups, sifted
- Bread machine yeast – 1 tsp.
- Fresh strawberries – 1 cup, chopped

Directions:

1. Place everything in the bread machine (except strawberries) according to the bread machine recommendations.
2. Select French bread and Medium crust.
3. Add the strawberries after the beep.
4. Remove the bread when done.
5. Cool, slice, and serve.

Nutrition Info: (Per Serving): Calories: 313; Total Fat: 0.9 g; Saturated Fat: 0.1 g; Carbohydrates: 65.7 g; Cholesterol: 0 mg; Fiber: 2.9 g; Calcium: 42 mg; Sodium: 973 mg; Protein: 9 g

Hot Cross Buns

Servings: 16 Bouns
Cooking Time: 10 Minutes Plus Fermenting Time
Ingredients:
- Dough
- 2 eggs plus enough water to equal 11/3 cups
- ½ cup butter, softened
- 4 cups bread flour
- ¾ teaspoon ground cinnamon
- ¼ teaspoon ground nutmeg
- 1½ teaspoons salt
- 2 tablespoons granulated sugar
- 1½ teaspoons bread machine or fast-acting dry yeast
- ½ cup raisins
- ½ cup golden raisins
- 1 egg
- 2 tablespoons cold water
- Icing
- 1 cup powdered sugar
- 1 tablespoon milk or water
- ½ teaspoon vanilla

Directions:
1. Preparing the Ingredients.
2. Measure carefully, placing all dough ingredients except raisins, 1 egg and the cold water in bread machine pan in the order recommended by the manufacturer. Add raisins at the Raisin/Nut signal.
3. Select the Bake cycle
4. Select Dough/Manual cycle. Do not use delay cycle. Remove dough from pan, using lightly floured hands. Cover and let rest 10 minutes on lightly floured surface. Grease cookie sheet or 2 (9-inch) round pans. Divide dough in half. Divide each half into 8 equal pieces. Shape each piece into a smooth ball. Place balls about 2 inches apart on cookie sheet or 1 inch apart in pans. Using scissors, snip a cross shape in top of each ball. Cover and let rise in warm place about 40 minutes or until doubled in size.
5. Heat oven to 375°F. Beat egg and cold water slightly; brush on buns. Bake 18 to 20 minutes or until golden brown. Remove from cookie sheet to cooling rack. Cool slightly.
6. In small bowl, mix all icing ingredients until smooth and spreadable. Make a cross on top of each bun with icing.

Buttery Sweet Bread

Servings: 1 Loaf
Cooking Time: 1 Hour And 15 Minutes
Ingredients:
- 1/3 cup water
- ½ cup milk
- ¼ cup of sugar
- One beaten egg
- One teaspoon of salt
- ¼ cup margarine or ¼ cup butter
- Two teaspoons bread machine yeast
- 3 1/3 cups bread flour

Directions:
1. Put everything in your bread machine pan.
2. Select the white bread setting.
3. Take out the pan when done and set aside for 10 minutes.

Nutrition Info: Calories 168;Carbohydrates: 28g;Total Fat 5g;Cholesterol 0mg;Protein 4g;Fiber 1g;Sugars 3g;Sodium 292mg;Potassium 50mg

Blue Cheese Bread

Servings: 12 Slices
Cooking Time: 10 Minutes
Ingredients:
- 3/4 cup warm water
- 1 large egg
- 1 teaspoon salt
- 3 cups bread flour
- 1 cup blue cheese, crumbled
- 2 tablespoons nonfat dry milk
- 2 tablespoons sugar

- 1 teaspoon bread machine yeast

Directions:

1. Preparing the Ingredients
2. Add the ingredients to bread machine pan in the order listed above, (except yeast) ; be sure to add the cheese with the flour.
3. Make a well in the flour; pour the yeast into the hole.
4. Select the Bake cycle
5. Select Basic bread cycle, medium crust color, and press Start.
6. When finished, transfer to a cooling rack for 10 minutes and serve warm.

Cheddar Cheese Bread

Servings: 20
Cooking Time: 3 Hours And 25 Minutes
Ingredients:

- Water – ¾ cup
- Egg – 1
- Salt – 1 tsp.
- Bread flour – 3 cups
- Shredded sharp cheddar cheese – 1 cup
- Nonfat dry milk – 2 tbsp.
- Sugar – 2 tbsp.
- Bread machine yeast – 1 tsp.

Directions:

1. Add everything according to bread machine recommendations.
2. Select Basic/White bread and Medium crust.
3. Remove the bread when done.
4. Cool, slice, and serve.

Nutrition Info: (Per Serving): Calories: 101; Total Fat: 2.3 g; Saturated Fat: 1.3 g; Carbohydrates: 15.8 g; Cholesterol: 15 mg; Fiber: 0.6 g; Calcium: 48 mg; Sodium: 157 mg; Protein: 3.8 g

Spinach And Feta Bread

Servings: 14 Slices
Cooking Time: 10 Minutes
Ingredients:

- 1 cup water
- 2 tsp butter
- 3 cups flour
- 1 tsp sugar

- 2 tsp instant minced onion
- 1 tsp salt
- 1¼ tsp instant yeast
- 1 cup crumbled feta
- 1 cup chopped fresh spinach leaves

Directions:

1. Preparing the Ingredients
2. Add each ingredient except the cheese and spinach to the bread machine in the order and at the temperature recommended by your bread machine manufacturer.
3. Select the Bake cycle
4. Close the lid, select the basic bread, medium crust setting on your bread machine, and press start.
5. When only 10 minutes are left in the last kneading cycle add the spinach and cheese.
6. When the bread machine has finished baking, remove the bread and put it on a cooling rack.

Apple Butter Bread

Servings: 1 Loaf
Cooking Time: 10 Minutes Plus Fermenting Time
Ingredients:

- 8 slices bread (1 pound)
- ⅔ cup milk, at 80°F to 90°F
- ⅓ cup apple butter, at room temperature
- 4 teaspoons melted butter, cooled
- 2 teaspoons honey
- ⅔ teaspoon salt
- ⅔ cup whole-wheat flour
- 1½ cups white bread flour
- 1 teaspoon bread machine or instant yeast

Directions:

1. Preparing the Ingredients.
2. Choose the size of loaf of your preference and then measure the ingredients.
3. Add all of the ingredients mentioned previously in the list.
4. Close the lid after placing the pan in the bread machine.
5. Select the Bake cycle
6. Turn on the bread machine. Select the Quick/Rapid setting, select the loaf size, and the crust color. Press start.
7. When the cycle is finished, carefully remove the pan from the bread maker and let it rest.

8. Remove the bread from the pan, put in a wire rack to Cool about 5 minutes. Slice

Double Cheese Bread

Servings: 8 Pcs
Cooking Time: 15 Minutes
Ingredients:
- ¾ cup plus one tablespoon milk, at 80°F to 90°F
- Two teaspoons butter, melted and cooled
- Four teaspoons sugar
- 2/3 teaspoon salt
- 1/3 teaspoon freshly ground black pepper
- Pinch cayenne pepper
- 1 cup (4 ounces) shredded aged sharp Cheddar cheese
- 1/3 cup shredded or grated Parmesan cheese
- 2 cups white bread flour
- ¾ teaspoon instant yeast

Directions:
1. Place the ingredients in your machine as recommended on it.
2. Make a program on the machine for Basic White bread, select light or medium crust, and press Start.
3. When the loaf is finished, remove the bucket from the machine.
4. Let the loaf cool for a minute.
5. Gently shake the bucket and remove the loaf and turn it out onto a rack to cool.
Nutrition Info: Calories: 183 calories;Total Carbohydrate: 28 g ;Total Fat: 4g ;Protein: 6 g ;Sodium: 344 mg

Ginger Spiced Bread

Servings: 1 Loaf
Ingredients:
- 16 slice bread (2 pounds)
- 1⅓ cups lukewarm buttermilk
- 1 egg, at room temperature
- ⅓ cup dark molasses
- 4 teaspoons unsalted butter, melted
- ¼ cup sugar
- 2 teaspoons table salt
- 4¼ cups white bread flour
- 2 teaspoons ground ginger
- 1¼ teaspoons ground cinnamon

- ⅔ teaspoon ground nutmeg
- ⅓ teaspoon ground cloves
- 2¼ teaspoons bread machine yeast
- 12 slice bread (1½ pounds)
- 1 cup lukewarm buttermilk
- 1 egg, at room temperature
- ¼ cup dark molasses
- 1 tablespoon unsalted butter, melted
- 3 tablespoons sugar
- 1½ teaspoons table salt
- 3½ cups white bread flour
- 1 teaspoon ground cinnamon
- ½ teaspoon ground nutmeg
- ¼ teaspoon ground cloves
- 1½ teaspoons ground ginger
- 2 teaspoons bread machine yeast

Directions:
1. Choose the size of loaf you would like to make and measure your ingredients.
2. Add the ingredients to the bread pan in the order listed above.
3. Place the pan in the bread machine and close the lid.
4. Turn on the bread maker. Select the Sweet setting, then the loaf size, and finally the crust color. Start the cycle.
5. When the cycle is finished and the bread is baked, carefully remove the pan from the machine. Use a potholder as the handle will be very hot. Let rest for a few minutes.
6. Remove the bread from the pan and allow to cool on a wire rack for at least 10 minutes before slicing.
Nutrition Info: (Per Serving):Calories 187, fat 2.3 g, carbs 36.7 g, sodium 312 mg, protein 4.6 g

Citrus Bread

Servings: 10
Cooking Time: 3 Hours And 25 Minutes
Ingredients:
- 1 whole egg
- Butter - 3 tbsp., melted
- White sugar - 1/3 cup
- Vanilla sugar - 1 tbsp.
- Tangerine juice - ½ cup

- Whole milk - 2/3 cup
- Kosher salt - 1 tsp.
- Bread machine flour - 4 cups
- Bread machine yeast - 1 tbsp.
- Candied oranges - ¼ cup
- Candied lemon - ¼ cup
- Lemon zest -2 tsp., finely grated
- Almonds - ¼ cup, chopped

Directions:
1. Add everything in the bread machine (except fruits, zest, and almonds) according to bread machine recommendations.
2. Select Basic/Sweetbread and Medium crust.
3. Add zest, fruits, and chopped almonds after the beep.
4. Remove the bread when done.
5. Cool, slice, and serve.

Nutrition Info: (Per Serving): Calories: 404; Total Fat: 9.1 g; Saturated Fat: 3.5 g; Carbohydrates: 71.5 g; Cholesterol: 34 mg; Fiber: 2.9 g; Calcium: 72 mg; Sodium: 345 mg; Protein: 9.8 g

Nectarine Cobbler Bread

Servings: 1 Loaf
Cooking Time: 10 Minutes Plus Fermenting Time /
Ingredients:
- 12 to 16 slice bread (1½ to 2 pounds)
- ½ cup (1 stick) butter, at room temperature
- 2 eggs, at room temperature
- 1 cup sugar
- ¼ cup milk, at room temperature
- 1 teaspoon pure vanilla extract
- 1 cup diced nectarines
- 1¾ cups all-purpose flour
- 1 teaspoon baking soda
- ½ teaspoon salt
- ½ teaspoon ground nutmeg
- ¼ teaspoon baking powder

Directions:
1. Preparing the Ingredients.
2. Place the butter, eggs, sugar, milk, vanilla, and nectarines in your bread machine.
3. Select the Bake cycle
4. Program the machine for Quick/Rapid bread and press Start.

5. While the wet ingredients are mixing, stir together the flour, baking soda, salt, nutmeg, and baking powder in a small bowl.
6. After the first fast mixing is done and the machine signals, add the dry ingredients.
7. When the cycle is finished, carefully remove the pan from the bread maker and let it rest.
8. Remove the bread from the pan, put in a wire rack to Cool about 10 minutes. Slice

Olive Cheese Bread

Servings: 8 Pcs
Cooking Time: 15 Minutes
Ingredients:
- 2/3 cup milk, set at 80°F to 90°F
- One tablespoon melted butter cooled
- 2/3 Teaspoon minced garlic
- One tablespoon sugar
- 2/3 teaspoon salt
- 2 cups white bread flour
- ½ cup (2 ounces) shredded Swiss cheese
- ¾ teaspoon bread machine or instant yeast
- ¼ cup chopped black olives

Directions:
1. Place the ingredients in your device as recommended on it.
2. Make a program on the machine for basic white Bread, select Light or medium crust, and press Start.
3. When the loaf is finished, remove the bucket from the machine.
4. Let the loaf cool for a minute.
5. Gently shake the bucket and remove the loaf and turn it out onto a rack to cool.

Nutrition Info: Calories: 175 calories;Total Carbohydrate: 27 g ;Total Fat: 5g ;Protein: 6 g ;Sodium: 260 mg

Apple Bread

Servings: 12
Cooking Time: 3 Hours And 25 Minutes
Ingredients:
- Bread machine yeast - 2½ tsp.
- Bread machine flour -3½ cups, sifted
- Sea salt - ½ tsp.
- Sugar - 6 tbsp.

- Vanillin - 1 bag
- Olive oil - 6 tbsp.
- Eggs - 3
- Lukewarm water - 1 cup
- Apples - 1 cup, peeled and diced

Directions:

1. Add everything according to bread machine recommendations.
2. Select Basic and Dark crust.
3. Remove the bread when done.
4. Cool, slice, and serve.

Nutrition Info: (Per Serving): Calories: 379; Total Fat: 12.5 g; Saturated Fat: 1.9 g; Carbohydrates: 59.1 g; Cholesterol: 61 mg; Fiber: 3.1 g; Calcium: 45 mg; Sodium: 173 mg; Protein: 8.4 g

Coconut Ginger Bread

Servings: 1 Loaf
Cooking Time: 1 Hour

Ingredients:

- 1 cup + 2 tbsp Half & Half
- One ¼ cup toasted shredded coconut
- Two large eggs
- ¼ cup oil
- 1 tsp coconut extract
- 1 tsp lemon extract
- 3/4 cup sugar
- 1 tbsp grated lemon peel
- 2 cups all-purpose flour
- 2 tbsp finely chopped candied ginger
- 1 tbsp baking powder
- ½ tsp salt
- One ¼ cup toasted shredded coconut

Directions:

1. Put everything in your bread machine pan.
2. Select the quick bread mode.
3. Press the start button.
4. Allow bread to cool on the wire rack until ready to serve (at least 20 minutes).

Nutrition Info: Calories 210;Carbohydrates: 45g;Total Fat 3g;Cholesterol3mg;Protein 5g;Fiber 2g;Sugar 15g;Sodium 185mg;Potassium 61mg

Tomato Cheese Bread

Servings: 8

Cooking Time: 3 Hours And 25 Minutes

Ingredients:

- Bread machine yeast - 1 tsp.
- Wheat bread flour - 2 ½ cups
- Sea salt - 1 ½ tsp.
- Sugar - 1 tbsp.
- Extra-virgin olive oil - 1 tbsp.
- Tomatoes - 5 tbsp. dried and filled with oil, chopped
- Parmesan cheese - ½ cup, grated
- Whole milk - 1 cup lukewarm

Directions:

1. Place all the ingredients (except tomatoes) in the pan according to bread machine recommendations.
2. Select Basic cycle and Medium crust.
3. Add the tomatoes after the beep.
4. Remove the bread when done.
5. Cool, slice, and serve.

Nutrition Info: (Per Serving): Calories: 209; Total Fat: 5.1 g; Saturated Fat: 2.2 g; Carbohydrates: 33.4 g; Cholesterol: 10 mg; Fiber: 1.2 g; Calcium: 42 mg; Sodium: 498 mg; Protein: 7 g

Apple Honey Bread

Servings: 1 Loaf
Cooking Time: 10 Minutes Plus Fermenting Time

Ingredients:

- 12 slice bread (1½ pounds)
- 5 tablespoons lukewarm milk
- 3 tablespoons apple cider, at room temperature
- 3 tablespoons sugar
- 2 tablespoons unsalted butter, melted
- 1½ tablespoons honey
- ¼ teaspoon table salt
- 3 cups white bread flour
- 1¼ teaspoons bread machine yeast
- 1 apple, peeled, cored, and finely diced

Directions:

1. Preparing the Ingredients.
2. Choose the size of loaf of your preference and then measure the ingredients.
3. Add all of the ingredients mentioned previously in the list, except for the apples. Close the lid after placing the pan in the bread machine.

4. Select the Bake cycle

5. Turn on the bread maker. Select the White/Basic or Fruit/Nut (if your machine has this setting) setting, then the loaf size, and finally the crust color. Start the cycle.

6. When the machine signals to add ingredients, add the apples. When the cycle is finished, carefully remove the pan from the bread maker and let it rest. Remove the bread from the pan, put in a wire rack to Cool about 5 minutes. Slice

Mozzarella And Salami Bread

Servings: 1 Loaf
Cooking Time: 10 Minutes Plus Fermenting Time
Ingredients:
- 12 slice bread (1½ pounds)
- 1 cup water plus 2 tablespoons, at 80°F to 90°F
- ½ cup (2 ounces) shredded mozzarella cheese
- 2 tablespoons sugar
- 1 teaspoon salt
- 1 teaspoon dried basil
- ¼ teaspoon garlic powder
- 3¼ cups white bread flour
- 1½ teaspoons bread machine or instant yeast
- ¾ cup finely diced hot German salami

Directions:
1. Preparing the Ingredients.
2. Place the ingredients, except the salami, in your bread machine as recommended by the manufacturer.
3. Program the machine for Basic/White bread, select light or medium crust, and press Start.
4. When the loaf is done, remove the bucket from the machine.
5. Select the Bake cycle
6. Add the salami when your machine signals or 5 minutes before the second kneading cycle is finished.
7. Let the loaf cool for 5 minutes. Gently shake the bucket to remove the loaf, and turn it out onto a rack to cool.

Feta Oregano Bread

Servings: 1 Loaf
Cooking Time: 10 Minutes Plus Fermenting Time
Ingredients:

- 8 slice bread (1 pounds)
- ⅔ cup milk, at 80°F to 90°F
- 2 teaspoons melted butter, cooled
- 2 teaspoons sugar
- ⅔ teaspoon salt
- 2 teaspoons dried oregano
- 2 cups white bread flour
- 1½ teaspoons bread machine or instant yeast
- ⅔ cup (2½ ounces) crumbled feta cheese

Directions:
1. Preparing the Ingredients.
2. Choose the size of loaf of your preference and then measure the ingredients.
3. Add all of the ingredients mentioned previously in the list.
4. Close the lid after placing the pan in the bread machine.
5. Select the Bake cycle
6. Turn on the bread machine. Select the Quick/Rapid setting, select the loaf size, and the crust color. Press start.
7. When the cycle is finished, carefully remove the pan from the bread maker and let it rest.
8. Remove the bread from the pan, put in a wire rack to Cool about 5 minutes. Slice

Coconut Delight Bread

Servings: 1 Loaf
Cooking Time: 10 Minutes Plus Fermenting Time
Ingredients:
- 16 slice bread (2 pounds)
- 1⅓ cups lukewarm milk
- 1 egg, at room temperature
- 2 tablespoons unsalted butter, melted
- 2⅔ teaspoons pure coconut extract
- 3⅓ tablespoons sugar
- 1 teaspoon table salt
- ⅔ cup sweetened shredded coconut
- 4 cups white bread flour
- 2 teaspoons bread machine yeast

Directions:
1. Preparing the Ingredients.
2. Choose the size of loaf of your preference and then measure the ingredients.

3. Add all of the ingredients mentioned previously in the list.
4. Close the lid after placing the pan in the bread machine.
5. Select the Bake cycle
6. Turn on the bread machine. Select the Sweet setting, select the loaf size, and the crust color. Press start.
7. When the cycle is finished, carefully remove the pan from the bread maker and let it rest.
8. Remove the bread from the pan, put in a wire rack to Cool about 5 minutes. Slice

Cranberry-cornmeal Bread

Servings: 1 Loaf
Cooking Time: 10 Minutes Plus Fermenting Time
Ingredients:
- 12 slice bread (1½ pounds)
- 1 cup plus 1 tablespoon water
- 3 tablespoons molasses or honey
- 2 tablespoons butter, softened
- 3 cups bread flour
- 1/3 cup cornmeal
- 1½ teaspoons salt
- 2 teaspoons bread machine yeast
- ½ cup sweetened dried cranberries

Directions:
1. Preparing the Ingredients.
2. Choose the size of loaf of your preference and then measure the ingredients.
3. Add all of the ingredients mentioned previously in the list except cranberries
4. Close the lid after placing the pan in the bread machine.
5. Add cranberries at the Raisin/Nut signal or 5 to 10 minutes before last kneading cycle ends.
6. Select the Bake cycle
7. Program the machine for White/Basic bread and press Start.
8. After the first fast mixing is done, add the flour, coconut, cinnamon, baking soda, baking powder, nutmeg, ginger, and allspice. When the cycle is finished, carefully remove the pan from the bread maker and let it rest.
9. Remove the bread from the pan, put in a wire rack to Cool about 5 minutes. Slice.

Basil Cheese Bread

Servings: 1 Loaf
Cooking Time: 10 Minutes Plus Fermenting Time
Ingredients:
- 12 slice bread (1½ pounds)
- 1 cup lukewarm milk
- 1 tablespoon unsalted butter, melted
- 1 tablespoon sugar
- 1 teaspoon dried basil
- ¾ teaspoon table salt
- ¾ cup sharp Cheddar cheese, shredded
- 3 cups white bread flour
- 1½ teaspoons bread machine yeast

Directions:
1. Preparing the Ingredients.
2. Choose the size of loaf of your preference and then measure the ingredients.
3. Add all of the ingredients mentioned previously in the list.
4. Close the lid after placing the pan in the bread machine.
5. Select the Bake cycle
6. Turn on the bread machine. Select the Quick/Rapid setting, select the loaf size, and the crust color. Press start.
7. When the cycle is finished, carefully remove the pan from the bread maker and let it rest.
8. Remove the bread from the pan, put in a wire rack to Cool about 5 minutes. Slice

Crunchy Wheat-and-honey Twist

Servings: 1 Loaf
Cooking Time: 10 Minutes Plus Fermenting Time
Ingredients:
- 16 slice bread (2 pounds)
- Bread dough
- ¾ cup plus 2 tablespoons water
- 2 tablespoons honey
- 1 tablespoon butter, softened
- 1¼ cups whole wheat flour
- 1 cup bread flour
- 1/3 cup slivered almonds, toasted
- 1 teaspoon salt

- 1 teaspoon bread machine or fast-acting dry yeast
- Topping
- Butter, melted
- 1 egg, slightly beaten
- 2 tablespoons sugar
- ¼ teaspoon ground cinnamon

Directions:

1. Preparing the Ingredients.
2. Measure carefully, placing all bread dough ingredients in bread machine pan in the order recommended by the manufacturer.
3. Select Dough/Manual cycle. Do not use delay cycle.
4. Remove dough from pan, using lightly floured hands. Cover and let rest 10 minutes on lightly floured surface.
5. Grease large cookie sheet with shortening. Divide dough in half. Roll each half into 15-inch rope. Place ropes side by side on cookie sheet; twist together gently and loosely. Pinch ends to seal. Brush melted butter lightly over dough.
6. Select the Bake cycle
7. Cover and let rise in warm place 45 to 60 minutes or until doubled in size.
8. Dough is ready if indentation remains when touched.
9. Heat oven to 375°F. Brush egg over dough. Mix sugar and cinnamon; sprinkle over dough. Bake 25 to 30 minutes or until twist is golden brown and sounds hollow when tapped. Remove from cookie sheet to cooling rack; cool 20 minutes.
10. To toast almonds, bake in ungreased shallow pan at 350°F for 6 to 10 minutes, stirring occasionally, until light brown.

Honey Granola Bread

Servings: 1 Loaf
Cooking Time: 10 Minutes Plus Fermenting Time
Ingredients:

- 12 slice bread (1½ pounds)
- 1⅛ cups milk, at 80°F to 90°F
- 3 tablespoons honey
- 1½ tablespoons butter, melted and cooled
- 1⅛ teaspoons salt
- ¾ cup whole-wheat flour

- ⅔ cup prepared granola, crushed
- 1¾ cups white bread flour
- 1½ teaspoons bread machine or instant yeast

Directions:

1. Preparing the Ingredients.
2. Choose the size of loaf of your preference and then measure the ingredients.
3. Add all of the ingredients mentioned previously in the list.
4. Close the lid after placing the pan in the bread machine.
5. Select the Bake cycle
6. Turn on the bread machine. Select the Basic/White setting, select the loaf size, and the crust color. Press start.
7. When the cycle is finished, carefully remove the pan from the bread maker and let it rest.
8. Remove the bread from the pan, put in a wire rack to Cool about 5 minutes. Slice

American Cheese Beer Bread

Servings: 1 Loaf
Ingredients:

- 16 slice bread (2 pounds)
- 1⅔ cups warm beer
- 1½ tablespoons sugar
- 2 teaspoons table salt
- 1½ tablespoons unsalted butter, melted
- ¾ cup American cheese, shredded
- ¾ cup Monterrey Jack cheese, shredded
- 4 cups white bread flour
- 2 teaspoons bread machine yeast
- 12 slice bread (1½ pounds)
- 1¼ cups warm beer
- 1 tablespoon sugar
- 1½ teaspoons table salt
- 1 tablespoon unsalted butter, melted
- ½ cup American cheese, shredded
- ½ cup Monterrey Jack cheese, shredded
- 3 cups white bread flour
- 1½ teaspoons bread machine yeast

Directions:

1. Choose the size of loaf you would like to make and measure your ingredients.

2. Add the ingredients to the bread pan in the order listed above.

3. Place the pan in the bread machine and close the lid.

4. Turn on the bread maker. Select the White/Basic setting, then the loaf size, and finally the crust color. Start the cycle.

5. When the cycle is finished and the bread is baked, carefully remove the pan from the machine. Use a potholder as the handle will be very hot. Let rest for a few minutes.

6. Remove the bread from the pan and allow to cool on a wire rack for at least 10 minutes before slicing.

Nutrition Info: (Per Serving):Calories 173, fat 5.3 g, carbs 26.1 g, sodium 118 mg, protein 6.2 g

Cheddar Cheese Basil Bread

Servings: 1 Loaf
Cooking Time: 10 Minutes
Ingredients:
- 12 slice bread (1½ pounds)
- 1 cup milk, at 80°F to 90°F
- 1 tablespoon melted butter, cooled
- 1 tablespoon sugar
- 1 teaspoon dried basil
- ¾ cup (3 ounces) shredded sharp Cheddar cheese
- ¾ teaspoon salt
- 3 cups white bread flour
- 1½ teaspoons bread machine or active dry yeast

Directions:

1. Preparing the Ingredients.

2. Choose the size of loaf of your preference and then measure the ingredients.

3. Add all of the ingredients mentioned previously in the list.

4. Close the lid after placing the pan in the bread machine.

5. Select the Bake cycle

6. Turn on the bread machine. Select the White/Basic setting, select the loaf size, and the crust color. Press start.

7. When the cycle is finished, carefully remove the pan from the bread maker and let it rest.

8. Remove the bread from the pan, put in a wire rack to Cool about 5 minutes. Slice

GLUTEN-FREE BREAD

Gluten-free Potato Bread

Servings: 12
Cooking Time: 3 Hours
Ingredients:
- 1 medium russet potato, baked, or mashed leftovers
- 2 packets gluten-free quick yeast
- 3 tablespoons honey
- 3/4 cup warm almond milk
- 2 eggs, 1 egg white
- 3 2/3 cups almond flour
- 3/4 cup tapioca flour
- 1 teaspoon sea salt
- 1 teaspoon dried chives
- 1 tablespoon apple cider vinegar
- 1/4 cup olive oil

Directions:
1. Combine all of the dry ingredients, except the yeast, in a large mixing bowl; set aside.
2. Whisk together the milk, eggs, oil, apple cider, and honey in a separate mixing bowl.
3. Pour the wet ingredients into the bread maker.
4. Add the dry ingredients on top of the wet ingredients.
5. Create a well in the dry ingredients and add the yeast.
6. Set to Gluten-Free bread setting, light crust color, and press Start.
7. Allow to cool completely before slicing.

Nutrition Info: Calories: 232, Sodium: 173 mg, Dietary Fiber: 6.3 g, Fat: 13.2 g, Carbs: 17.4 g, Protein: 10.4 g.

Gluten-free Pizza Crust

Servings: 6 - 8
Cooking Time: 2 Hours
Ingredients:
- 3 large eggs, room temperature
- 1/2 cup olive oil
- 1 cup milk
- 1/2 cup water
- 2 cups rice flour
- 1 cup cornstarch, and extra for dusting
- 1/2 cup potato starch
- 1/2 cup sugar
- 2 tablespoons yeast
- 3 teaspoons xanthan gum
- 1 teaspoon salt

Directions:
1. Combine the wet ingredients in a separate bowl and pour into the bread maker pan.
2. Combine the dry ingredients except yeast and add to pan.
3. Make a well in the center of the dry ingredients and add the yeast.
4. Select Dough cycle and press Start.
5. When dough is finished, press it out on a surface lightly sprinkled with corn starch and create a pizza shape. Use this dough with your favorite toppings and pizza recipe!

Nutrition Info: Calories: 463, Sodium: 547 mg, Dietary Fiber: 8.1 g, Fat: 15.8 g, Carbs: 79.2 g, Protein: 7.4 g.

Grain-free Chia Bread

Servings: 12
Cooking Time: 3 Hours
Ingredients:
- 1 cup warm water
- 3 large organic eggs, room temperature
- 1/4 cup olive oil
- 1 tablespoon apple cider vinegar
- 1 cup gluten-free chia seeds, ground to flour
- 1 cup almond meal flour
- 1/2 cup potato starch
- 1/4 cup coconut flour
- 3/4 cup millet flour
- 1 tablespoon xanthan gum
- 1 1/2 teaspoons salt
- 2 tablespoons sugar
- 3 tablespoons nonfat dry milk
- 6 teaspoons instant yeast

Directions:
1. Whisk wet ingredients together and add to the bread maker pan.
2. Whisk dry ingredients, except yeast, together and add on top of wet ingredients.

3.	Make a well in the dry ingredients and add yeast.
4.	Select Whole Wheat cycle, light crust color, and press Start.
5.	Allow to cool completely before serving.
Nutrition Info: Calories: 375, Sodium: 462 mg, Dietary Fiber: 22.3 g, Fat: 18.3 g, Carbs: 42 g, Protein: 12.2 g.

Italian Parmesan Cheese Bread

Servings: 6 Pcs.
Cooking Time: 1 Hour
Ingredients:
- 300ml (1 ¼ cups) warm water
- 60ml (¼ cup) olive oil
- Two egg whites
- One tablespoon apple cider vinegar
- ½ teaspoon baking powder
- 7g (2 teaspoons) dry active yeast
- Two tablespoons granulated sugar
- 200g (2 cups) gluten-free almond flour / or any other gluten-free flour, levelled
- 100g (1 cup) Tapioca/potato starch, levelled
- Two teaspoons Xanthan Gum
- 28g (¼ cup) grated Parmesan cheese
- One teaspoon salt
- One teaspoon Italian seasoning
- One teaspoon garlic powder

Directions:
1.	According to your bread machine manufacturer, place all the ingredients into the bread machine's greased pan and select a basic cycle / standard cycle/bake / quick bread / white bread setting. Then choose crust colour, either medium or light and press start to bake bread.
2.	In the last kneading cycle, check the dough
3.	it should be wet but thick, not like traditional bread dough. If the dough is too wet, put more flour, one tablespoon at a time, or until dough slightly firm.
4.	When the cycle is finished and the machine turns off, remove baked bread from pan and cool on wire rack.
Nutrition Info: Calories: 90 Calories;Total fat: 2 g;Cholesterol: 2 mg;Sodium: 48 mg;Carbohydrates: 15g;Fibre: 1 g;Protein: 2 g

Gluten-free Simple Sandwich Bread

Servings: 12
Cooking Time: 1 Hour
Ingredients:
- 1 1/2 cups sorghum flour
- 1 cup tapioca starch or potato starch (not potato flour!)
- 1/2 cup gluten-free millet flour or gluten-free oat flour
- 2 teaspoons xanthan gum
- 1 1/4 teaspoons fine sea salt
- 2 1/2 teaspoons gluten-free yeast for bread machines
- 1 1/4 cups warm water
- 3 tablespoons extra virgin olive oil
- 1 tablespoon honey or raw agave nectar
- 1/2 teaspoon mild rice vinegar or lemon juice
- 2 organic free-range eggs, beaten

Directions:
1.	Whisk together the dry ingredients except the yeast and set aside.
2.	Add the liquid ingredients to the bread maker pan first, then gently pour the mixed dry ingredients on top of the liquid.
3.	Make a well in the center of the dry ingredients and add the yeast.
4.	Set for Rapid 1 hour 20 minutes, medium crust color, and press Start.
5.	Transfer to a cooling rack for 15 minutes before slicing to serve.
Nutrition Info: Calories: 137, Sodium: 85 mg, Dietary Fiber: 2.7 g, Fat: 4.6 g, Carbs: 22.1 g, Protein: 2.4 g.

Easy Gluten-free, Dairy-free Bread

Servings: 12
Cooking Time: 2 Hours 10 Minutes
Ingredients:
- 1 1/2 cups warm water
- 2 teaspoons active dry yeast
- 2 teaspoons sugar
- 2 eggs, room temperature
- 1 egg white, room temperature
- 1 1/2 tablespoons apple cider vinegar
- 4 1/2 tablespoons olive oil

- 3 1/3 cups multi-purpose gluten-free flour

Directions:

1. Add the yeast and sugar to the warm water and stir to mix in a large mixing bowl; set aside until foamy, about 8 to 10 minutes.
2. Whisk the 2 eggs and 1 egg white together in a separate mixing bowl and add to baking pan of bread maker.
3. Add apple cider vinegar and oil to baking pan.
4. Add foamy yeast/water mixture to baking pan.
5. Add the multi-purpose gluten-free flour on top.
6. Set for Gluten-Free bread setting and Start.
7. Remove and invert pan onto a cooling rack to remove the bread from the baking pan. Allow to cool completely before slicing to serve.

Nutrition Info: Calories: 241, Sodium: 164 mg, Dietary Fiber: 5.6 g, Fat: 6.8 g, Carbs: 41 g, Protein: 4.5 g.

Gluten-free Sourdough Bread

Servings: 12
Cooking Time: 3 Hours
Ingredients:

- 1 cup water
- 3 eggs
- 3/4 cup ricotta cheese
- 1/4 cup honey
- 1/4 cup vegetable oil
- 1 teaspoon cider vinegar
- 3/4 cup gluten-free sourdough starter
- 2 cups white rice flour
- 2/3 cup potato starch
- 1/3 cup tapioca flour
- 1/2 cup dry milk powder
- 3 1/2 teaspoons xanthan gum
- 1 1/2 teaspoons salt

Directions:

1. Combine wet ingredients and pour into bread maker pan.
2. Mix together dry ingredients in a large mixing bowl, and add on top of the wet ingredients.
3. Select Gluten-Free cycle and press Start.
4. Remove the pan from the machine and allow the bread to remain in the pan for approximately 10 minutes.
5. Transfer to a cooling rack before slicing.

Nutrition Info: Calories: 299, Sodium: 327 mg, Dietary Fiber: 1.0 g, Fat: 7.3 g, Carbs: 46 g, Protein: 5.2 g.

Gluten-free Cinnamon Raisin Bread

Servings: 12
Cooking Time: 3 Hours
Ingredients:

- 3/4 cup almond milk
- 2 tablespoons flax meal
- 6 tablespoons warm water
- 1 1/2 teaspoons apple cider vinegar
- 2 tablespoons butter
- 1 1/2 tablespoons honey
- 1 2/3 cups brown rice flour
- 1/4 cup corn starch
- 2 tablespoons potato starch
- 1 1/2 teaspoons xanthan gum
- 1 tablespoon cinnamon
- 1/2 teaspoon salt
- 1 teaspoon active dry yeast
- 1/2 cup raisins

Directions:

1. Mix together flax and water and let stand for 5 minutes.
2. Combine dry ingredients in a separate bowl, except for yeast.
3. Add wet ingredients to the bread machine.
4. Add the dry mixture on top and make a well in the middle of the dry mixture.
5. Add the yeast to the well.
6. Set to Gluten Free, light crust color, and press Start.
7. After first kneading and rise cycle, add raisins.
8. Remove to a cooling rack when baked and let cool for 15 minutes before slicing.

Nutrition Info: Calories: 192, Sodium: 173 mg, Dietary Fiber: 4.4 g, Fat: 4.7 g, Carbs: 38.2 g, Protein: 2.7 g.

Paleo Bread

Servings: 16
Cooking Time: 3 Hours 15 Minutes
Ingredients:

- 4 tablespoons chia seeds

- 1 tablespoon flax meal
- 3/4 cup, plus 1 tablespoon water
- 1/4 cup coconut oil
- 3 eggs, room temperature
- 1/2 cup almond milk
- 1 tablespoon honey
- 2 cups almond flour
- 1 1/4 cups tapioca flour
- 1/3 cup coconut flour
- 1 teaspoon salt
- 1/4 cup flax meal
- 2 teaspoons cream of tartar
- 1 teaspoon baking soda
- 2 teaspoons active dry yeast

Directions:

1. Combine the chia seeds and tablespoon of flax meal in a mixing bowl; stir in the water and set aside.
2. Melt the coconut oil in a microwave-safe dish, and let it cool down to lukewarm.
3. Whisk in the eggs, almond milk and honey.
4. Whisk in the chia seeds and flax meal gel and pour it into the bread maker pan.
5. Stir the almond flour, tapioca flour, coconut flour, salt and 1/4 cup of flax meal together.
6. Mix the cream of tartar and baking soda in a separate bowl and combine it with the other dry ingredients.
7. Pour the dry ingredients into the bread machine.
8. Make a little well on top and add the yeast.
9. Start the machine on the Wheat cycle, light or medium crust color, and press Start.
10. Remove to cool completely before slicing to serve.

Nutrition Info: Calories: 190, Sodium: 243 mg, Dietary Fiber: 5.2 g, Fat: 10.3 g, Carbs: 20.4 g, Protein: 4.5 g.

Sandwich Bread

Servings: 1 Loaf (16 Slices).
Cooking Time: 1 Hour
Ingredients:

- 1 tbsp. active dry yeast
- 2 tbsps. sugar
- 1 cup warm fat-free milk (110° to 115°)
- Two eggs

- 3 tbsps. canola oil
- 1 tsp. cider vinegar
- 2-1/2 cups gluten-free all-purpose baking flour
- 2-1/2 tsp. xanthan gum
- 1 tsp. unflavored gelatin
- 1/2 tsp. salt

Directions:

1. Oil a loaf pan, 9x5 inches in size, and dust with gluten-free flour reserve.
2. In warm milk, melt sugar and yeast in a small bowl—mix yeast mixture, vinegar, oil, and eggs in a stand with a paddle. Slowly whip in salt, gelatin, xanthan gum and flour. Whip for a minute on low speed. Whip for 2 minutes on moderate. The dough will become softer compared to the yeast bread dough that has gluten. Turn onto the prepped pan. Using a wet spatula, smoothen the surface. Put a cover and rise in a warm area for 25 minutes until dough extends to the pan top.
3. Bake for 20 minutes at 375°
4. loosely cover with foil. Bake till golden brown for 10 to 15 minutes more. Take out from pan onto a wire rack to let cool.

Nutrition Info: Calories: 110 calories;Total Carbohydrate: 17 g;Cholesterol: 27 mg;Total Fat: 4 g;Fiber: 2 g;Protein: 4 g;Sodium: 95 mg

Gluten-free Whole Grain Bread

Servings: 12
Cooking Time: 3 Hours 40 Minutes
Ingredients:

- 2/3 cup sorghum flour
- 1/2 cup buckwheat flour
- 1/2 cup millet flour
- 3/4 cup potato starch
- 2 1/4 teaspoons xanthan gum
- 1 1/4 teaspoons salt
- 3/4 cup skim milk
- 1/2 cup water
- 1 tablespoon instant yeast
- 5 teaspoons agave nectar, separated
- 1 large egg, lightly beaten
- 4 tablespoons extra virgin olive oil
- 1/2 teaspoon cider vinegar
- 1 tablespoon poppy seeds

Directions:

1. Whisk sorghum, buckwheat, millet, potato starch, xanthan gum, and sea salt in a bowl and set aside.
2. Combine milk and water in a glass measuring cup. Heat to between 110°F and 120°F; add 2 teaspoons of agave nectar and yeast and stir to combine. Cover and set aside for a few minutes.
3. Combine the egg, olive oil, remaining agave, and vinegar in another mixing bowl; add yeast and milk mixture. Pour wet ingredients into the bottom of your bread maker.
4. Top with dry ingredients.
5. Select Gluten-Free cycle, light color crust, and press Start.
6. After second kneading cycle sprinkle with poppy seeds.
7. Remove pan from bread machine. Leave the loaf in the pan for about 5 minutes before cooling on a rack.
8. Enjoy!

Nutrition Info: Calories: 153, Sodium: 346 mg, Dietary Fiber: 4.1 g, Fat: 5.9 g, Carbs: 24.5 g, Protein: 3.3 g.

Cinnamon Raisin Bread

Servings: 1 Loaf (12 Slices)
Cooking Time: 1 Hour
Ingredients:

- 300ml (1 ¼ cups) warm water
- 60ml (¼ cup) olive oil
- Two tablespoons honey
- Two egg whites
- One tablespoon apple cider vinegar
- ½ teaspoon baking powder
- 7g (2 teaspoons) dry active yeast
- Two tablespoons granulated sugar
- 200g (2 cups) gluten-free almond flour / or any other gluten-free flour, levelled
- 100g (1 cup) Tapioca/potato starch, levelled
- Two teaspoons Xanthan Gum
- One teaspoon salt
- One teaspoon ground cinnamon
- 150g (1 cup) raisins

Directions:

1. According to your bread machine manufacturer, place all the ingredients into the bread machine's greased pan except raisins.
2. Select basic cycle / standard cycle/bake / quick bread / sweet bread setting
3. then choose crust colour either medium or Light and press start to bake bread.
4. In the last kneading cycle, check the dough
5. it should be wet but thick, not like traditional bread dough. If the dough is too wet, put more flour, one tablespoon at a time, or until dough slightly firm.
6. Add raisins 5 minutes before the kneading cycle ends.
7. When the cycle is finished and the machine turns off, remove baked bread from pan and cool on wire rack.

Nutrition Info: Calories: 89 Calories;Fat: 1 g;Cholesterol: 2 mg;Sodium: 10 mg;Carbohydrates: 12 g

Flax And Sunflower Seeds Bread

Servings: 8 Pcs
Cooking Time: 1 Hour
Ingredients:

- 300ml (1 ¼ cups) warm water
- 60ml (¼ cup) olive oil
- Two egg whites
- One tablespoon apple cider vinegar
- ½ teaspoon baking powder
- 7g (2 teaspoons) dry active yeast
- Two tablespoons granulated sugar
- 200g (2 cups) gluten-free almond flour / or any other gluten-free flour, levelled
- 100g (1 cup) Tapioca/potato starch, levelled
- Two teaspoons Xanthan Gum
- One teaspoon salt
- 55g (½ cup) flax seeds
- 55g (½ cup) sunflower seeds

Directions:

1. According to your bread machine manufacturer, place all the ingredients into the bread machine's greased pan except sunflower seeds.
2. Select basic cycle / standard cycle/bake / quick bread / white bread setting
3. then select crust colour either medium or light and press start.

4. In the last kneading cycle, check the dough

5. it should be wet but thick, not like traditional bread dough. If the dough is too wet, put more flour, one tablespoon at a time, or until dough slightly firm.

6. Add sunflower seeds 5 minutes before the kneading cycle ends.

7. When the cycle is finished and the machine turns off, remove baked bread from pan and cool on wire rack.

Nutrition Info: Calories: 90 Calories;Total fat: 2g;Cholesterol: 5 mg;Sodium: 180 mg;Carbohydrates: 18 g;Fibre: 2 g;Protein: 4 g

Sorghum Bread Recipe

Servings: 12
Cooking Time: 3 Hours
Ingredients:
- 1 1/2 cups sorghum flour
- 1 cup tapioca starch
- 1/2 cup brown or white sweet rice flour
- 1 teaspoon xanthan gum
- 1 teaspoon guar gum
- 1/2 teaspoon salt
- 3 tablespoons sugar
- 2 1/4 teaspoons instant yeast
- 3 eggs (room temperature, lightly beaten)
- 1/4 cup oil
- 1 1/2 teaspoons vinegar
- 3/4-1 cup milk (105 - 115°F)

Directions:
1. Combine the dry ingredients in a mixing bowl, except for yeast.

2. Add the wet ingredients to the bread maker pan, then add the dry ingredients on top.

3. Make a well in the center of the dry ingredients and add the yeast.

4. Set to Basic bread cycle, light crust color, and press Start.

5. Remove and lay on its side to cool on a wire rack before serving.

Nutrition Info: Calories: 169, Sodium: 151 mg, Dietary Fiber: 2.5 g, Fat: 6.3 g, Carbs: 25.8 g, Protein: 3.3 g.

Gluten-free Brown Bread

Servings: 12
Cooking Time: 3 Hours
Ingredients:
- 2 large eggs, lightly beaten
- 1 3/4 cups warm water
- 3 tablespoons canola oil
- 1 cup brown rice flour
- 3/4 cup oat flour
- 1/4 cup tapioca starch
- 1 1/4 cups potato starch
- 1 1/2 teaspoons salt
- 2 tablespoons brown sugar
- 2 tablespoons gluten-free flaxseed meal
- 1/2 cup nonfat dry milk powder
- 2 1/2 teaspoons xanthan gum
- 3 tablespoons psyllium, whole husks
- 2 1/2 teaspoons gluten-free yeast for bread machines

Directions:
1. Add the eggs, water and canola oil to the bread maker pan and stir until combined.

2. Whisk all of the dry ingredients except the yeast together in a large mixing bowl.

3. Add the dry ingredients on top of the wet ingredients.

4. Make a well in the center of the dry ingredients and add the yeast.

5. Set Gluten-Free cycle, medium crust color, and press Start.

6. When the bread is done, lay the pan on its side to cool before slicing to serve.

Nutrition Info: Calories: 201, Sodium: 390 mg, Dietary Fiber: 10.6 g, Fat: 5.7 g, Carbs: 35.5 g, Protein: 5.1 g.

Gluten-free Pumpkin Pie Bread

Servings: 12
Cooking Time: 2 Hours 50 Minutes
Ingredients:
- 1/4 cup olive oil
- 2 large eggs, beaten
- 1 tablespoon bourbon vanilla extract
- 1 cup canned pumpkin
- 4 tablespoons honey

- 1/4 teaspoon lemon juice
- 1/2 cup buckwheat flour
- 1/4 cup millet flour
- 1/4 cup sorghum flour
- 1/2 cup tapioca starch
- 1 cup light brown sugar
- 2 teaspoons baking powder
- 1 teaspoon baking soda
- 1/2 teaspoon sea salt
- 1 teaspoon xanthan gum
- 1 teaspoon ground cinnamon
- 1 teaspoon allspice
- 1-2 tablespoons peach juice

Directions:

1. Mix dry ingredients together in a bowl and put aside.
2. Add wet ingredients to pan, except peach juice.
3. Add mixed dry ingredients to bread maker pan.
4. Set to Sweet bread cycle, light or medium crust color, and press Start.
5. As it begins to mix the ingredients, use a soft silicone spatula to scrape down the sides.
6. If the batter is stiff, add one tablespoon at a time of peach juice until the batter becomes slightly thinner than muffin batter.
7. Close the lid and allow to bake. Remove to a cooling rack for 20 minutes before slicing.

Nutrition Info: Calories: 180, Sodium: 229 mg, Dietary Fiber: 2.5 g, Fat: 5.5 g, Carbs: 33.1 g, Protein: 2.4 g.

Gluten-free Pull-apart Rolls

Servings: 9
Cooking Time: 2 Hours
Ingredients:
- 1 cup warm water
- 2 tablespoons butter, unsalted
- 1 egg, room temperature
- 1 teaspoon apple cider vinegar
- 2 3/4 cups gluten-free almond-blend flour
- 1 1/2 teaspoons xanthan gum
- 1/4 cup sugar
- 1 teaspoon salt
- 2 teaspoons active dry yeast

Directions:

1. Add wet ingredients to the bread maker pan.
2. Mix dry ingredients except for yeast, and put in pan.
3. Make a well in the center of the dry ingredients and add the yeast.
4. Select Dough cycle and press Start.
5. Spray an 8-inch round cake pan with non-stick cooking spray.
6. When Dough cycle is complete, roll dough out into 9 balls, place in cake pan, and baste each with warm water.
7. Cover with a towel and let rise in a warm place for 1 hour.
8. Preheat oven to 400°F.
9. Bake for 26 to 28 minutes; until golden brown.
10. Brush with butter and serve.

Nutrition Info: Calories: 568, Sodium: 380 mg, Dietary Fiber: 5.5 g, Fat: 10.5 g, Carbs: 116.3 g, Protein: 8.6 g.

Gluten-free Crusty Boule Bread

Servings: 12
Cooking Time: 3 Hours
Ingredients:
- 3 1/4 cups gluten-free flour mix
- 1 tablespoon active dry yeast
- 1 1/2 teaspoons kosher salt
- 1 tablespoon guar gum
- 1 1/3 cups warm water
- 2 large eggs, room temperature
- 2 tablespoons, plus 2 teaspoons olive oil
- 1 tablespoon honey

Directions:

1. Combine all of the dry ingredients, except the yeast, in a large mixing bowl; set aside.
2. Whisk together the water, eggs, oil, and honey in a separate mixing bowl.
3. Pour the wet ingredients into the bread maker.
4. Add the dry ingredients on top of the wet ingredients.
5. Make a well in the center of the dry ingredients and add the yeast.
6. Set to Gluten-Free setting and press Start.
7. Remove baked bread and allow to cool completely. Hollow out and fill with soup or dip to use as a boule, or slice for serving.

Nutrition Info: Calories: 480, Sodium: 490 mg, Dietary Fiber: 67.9 g, Fat: 3.2 g, Carbs: 103.9 g, Protein: 2.4 g.

Gluten-free Oat & Honey Bread

Servings: 12
Cooking Time: 3 Hours
Ingredients:

- 1 1/4 cups warm water
- 3 tablespoons honey
- 2 eggs
- 3 tablespoons butter, melted
- 1 1/4 cups gluten-free oats
- 1 1/4 cups brown rice flour
- 1/2 cup potato starch
- 2 teaspoons xanthan gum
- 1 1/2 teaspoons sugar
- 3/4 teaspoon salt
- 1 1/2 tablespoons active dry yeast

Directions:

1. Add ingredients in the order listed above, except for yeast.
2. Make a well in the center of the dry ingredients and add the yeast.
3. Select Gluten-Free cycle, light crust color, and press Start.
4. Remove bread and allow the bread to cool on its side on a cooling rack for 20 minutes before slicing to serve.

Nutrition Info: Calories: 151, Sodium: 265 mg, Dietary Fiber: 4.3 g, Fat: 4.5 g, Carbs: 27.2 g, Protein: 3.5 g.

Cheese & Herb Bread

Servings: 1 Loaf (12 Slices)

Cooking Time: 1 Hour
Ingredients:

- 300ml (1 ¼ cups) warm water
- 60ml (¼ cup) olive oil
- Two egg whites
- One tablespoon apple cider vinegar
- ½ teaspoon baking powder
- 7g (2 teaspoons) dry active yeast
- Two tablespoons granulated sugar
- 200g (2 cups) gluten-free almond flour / or any other gluten-free flour, levelled
- 100g (1 cup) Tapioca/potato starch, levelled
- Two teaspoons Xanthan Gum
- One teaspoon salt
- Two tablespoons grated Parmesan cheese
- One teaspoon dried marjoram
- ¾ teaspoon dried basil
- ¾ teaspoon dried oregano

Directions:

1. According to your bread machine manufacturer, place all the ingredients into the bread machine's greased pan, and select a basic cycle / standard cycle/bake / quick bread / white bread setting. Then choose crust colour, either medium or light, and press start to bake bread.
2. In the last kneading cycle, check the dough
3. it should be wet but thick, not like traditional bread dough. If the dough is too wet, put more flour, one tablespoon at a time, or until dough slightly firm.
4. When the cycle is finished and the machine turns off, remove baked bread from pan and cool on wire rack.

Nutrition Info: Calories: 150 Calories;Total fat: 3 g;Cholesterol: 5 mg;Sodium: 415 mg;Carbohydrates: 9 g;Fibre: 1 g;Protein: 4 g

BREAD FROM AROUND THE WORLD

Sauerkraut Bread

Servings: 1 Loaf (22 Slices)
Cooking Time: 1 Hour And 30 Minutes
Ingredients:
- 1 cup lukewarm water (80 degrees F)
- ¼ cup cabbage brine
- ½ cup finely chopped cabbage
- Two tablespoons sunflower oil
- Two teaspoons white sugar
- 1½ teaspoons salt
- 2 1/3 cups rye flour
- 2 1/3 cups wheat flour
- Two teaspoons dry kvass
- Two teaspoons active dry yeast

Directions:
1. Prepare all of the ingredients for your bread and measuring means (a cup, a spoon, kitchen scales).
2. Finely chop the sauerkraut.
3. Carefully measure the ingredients into the pan.
4. Place all of the ingredients into a bucket in the right order, follow your manual bread machine.
5. Close the cover.
6. Select the program of your bread machine to BASIC and choose the crust colour to DARK.
7. Press START.
8. Wait until the program completes.
9. When done, take the bucket out and let it cool for 5-10 minutes.
10. Shake the loaf from the pan and let cool for 30 minutes on a cooling rack.
11. Slice, serve and enjoy the taste of fragrant homemade bread.

Nutrition Info: Calories 297;Total Fat 4.9g;Saturated Fat 0.5g;Cholesterol 0g;Sodium 442mg;Total Carbohydrate 55.5g;Dietary Fiber 9.7g;Total Sugars 1.6g;Protein 9.5g

Rye Bread With Caraway

Servings: 1 Pound Loaf
Cooking Time: 4 Hours
Ingredients:
- Lukewarm water :¾ cup
- Unsalted butter, diced :1 tbsp
- Molasses :1 tbsp
- Rye flour :½ cup
- Plain bread flour :1 cup
- Whole wheat flour :½ cup
- Milk powder :1 tbsp
- Salt :¾ tsp
- Brown sugar :2 tbsp
- Caraway seeds :1 tbsp
- Instant dry yeast :1 ¼ tsp

Directions:
1. Add the ingredients into the bread machine as per the order of the ingredients listed above or follow your bread machine's instruction manual.
2. Select the whole wheat setting and medium crust function.
3. When ready, turn the bread out onto a drying rack and allow it to cool, then serve.

Nutrition Info: (Per Serving):Calories: 93 kcal / Total fat: 2.3 g / Saturated fat: 1.3 g / Cholesterol: 5 mg / Total carbohydrates: 16.5 g / Dietary fiber: 2.3 g / Sodium: 218 mg / Protein: 2.4 g

Mexican Sweetbread

Servings: 12
Cooking Time: 3 Hours And 25 Minutes
Ingredients:
- Milk – 1 cup
- Butter – ¼ cup
- Egg – 1
- Sugar – ¼ cup
- Salt – 1 tsp.
- Bread flour – 3 cups
- Yeast – 1 ½ tsp.

Directions:
1. Place all ingredients in the bread machine according to bread machine recommendations.
2. Select Basic or Sweet cycle. Press Start.
3. Remove the bread when done.
4. Cool, slice, and serve.

Nutrition Info: (Per Serving): Calories: 184.3; Total Fat: 5.3 g; Saturated Fat: 1.3 g; Carbohydrates: 29.2 g; Cholesterol: 20.5 mg; Fiber: 0.9 g; Calcium: 38 mg; Sodium: 254.8 mg; Protein: 4.7 g

Keto Focaccia Bread

Servings: 1 Loaf
Cooking Time: 23-30 Minutes
Ingredients:
- 1 cup almond flour
- 1/3 cup coconut flour
- 1/3 cup protein powder, unflavored and unsweetened
- Two tablespoons rosemary, chopped
- One tablespoon baking powder
- ¾ teaspoon salt
- ½ teaspoon garlic powder
- Two eggs, whole
- Two egg whites
- ½ cup extra-virgin olive oil
- ½ cup of water

Directions:
1. Place the wet ingredients first in the bread pan, followed by the dry ingredients.
2. Set the bread machine to "Manual" or "Dough" mode.
3. Once the cycles are completed, put the dough on a surface with a light dusting of flour.
4. Shape the dough into a ball.
5. Flatten the dough on a greased baking sheet until it becomes a 10-inch circle.
6. Cover the dough, and allow it to rise for 15 minutes.
7. Preheat the oven to 375F.
8. Bake for 25 to 30 minutes.
Nutrition Info: Calories: 174 Cal;Carbohydrates: 5 g;Fat: 15g

Honey And Milk White Bread

Servings: 1 Pound Loaf
Cooking Time: 3 Hours
Ingredients:
- Lukewarm whole milk :½ cup
- Unsalted butter :¾ tbsp
- Honey :¾ tbsp
- White all-purpose Flour :1 ½ cups
- Salt :1 pinch
- Bread machine yeast :2/4 tsp

Directions:

1. Add the ingredients into the bread machine as per the order of the ingredients listed above or follow your bread machine's instruction manual.
2. Select the white bread function and the light crust function.
3. When ready, turn the bread out onto a drying rack and allow it to cool, then serve.
Nutrition Info: (Per Serving):Calories: 102.5 kcal / Total fat: 1.9 g / Saturated fat: 0.7 g / Cholesterol: 2.4 mg / Total carbohydrates: 18.3 g / Dietary fiber: 0.7 g / Sodium: 202.8 mg / Protein: 2.9 g

Keto Breadsticks

Servings: 2 Pcs
Cooking Time: 15-20 Minutes
Ingredients:
- 1 ½ cup mozzarella cheese, shredded
- 1-ounce cream cheese
- ½ cup almond flour
- Three tablespoons coconut flour
- One egg
- ½ cup mozzarella cheese, shredded
- 1/3 cup parmesan cheese, shredded
- ¼ cup egg wash
- One teaspoon parsley, finely chopped

Directions:
1. Add the ingredients for the bread into the bread pan.
2. Put the bread machine on "Manual" or "Dough" mode.
3. After the cycles are finished, place the dough on a surface with a light dusting of flour.
4. Divide the dough into four and then divide each quarter again into 6.
5. Roll each piece until it is 8 inches long. Place the rolled dough on a greased baking sheet.
6. Brush over each piece with the egg wash.
7. Cover, and allow it to rise for 10 minutes.
8. Preheat the oven t0 4000F.
9. Spread half of the toppings on each piece.
10. Bake for 5 minutes before spreading the remaining toppings on the breadsticks.
11. Bake for another 10 minutes, or until the cheese has melted.
12. Remove it and then let it cool down on a wire rack.

Nutrition Info: Calories: 207;Carbohydrates: 7g;Fat: 14g;Protein: 13g

Italian Bread

Servings: 2 Loaves
Cooking Time: 1 Hour And 10 Minutes
Ingredients:
- One tablespoon of light brown sugar
- 4 cups all-purpose flour, unbleached
- 1 ½ teaspoon of salt
- One 1/3 cups + 1 tablespoon warm water
- One package active dry yeast
- 1 ½ teaspoon of olive oil
- One egg
- Two tablespoons cornmeal

Directions:
1. Place flour, brown sugar, 1/3 cup warm water, salt, olive oil, and yeast in your bread machine. Select the dough cycle. Hit the start button.
2. Deflate your dough. Turn it on a floured surface.
3. Form two loaves from the dough.
4. Keep them on your cutting board. The seam side should be down. Sprinkle some cornmeal on your board.
5. Place a damp cloth on your loaves to cover them.
6. Wait for 40 minutes. The volume should double.
7. In the meantime, preheat your oven to 190 °C.
8. Beat 1 tablespoon of water and an egg in a bowl.
9. Brush this mixture on your loaves.
10. Make an extended cut at the center of your loaves with a knife.
11. Shake your cutting board gently, making sure that the loaves do not stick.
12. Now slide your loaves on a baking sheet.
13. Bake in your oven for about 35 minutes.
Nutrition Info: Calories 105;Carbohydrates: 20.6 g;Total Fat 0.9;Cholesterol 9 mg;Protein 3.1 g;Fiber 1 g;Sugar 1g;Sodium 179 mg;Potassium 39 mg

Pizza Dough Recipe

Servings: 6 Servings
Cooking Time: 1 Hour And 30 Minutes
Ingredients:
- ● 2 cups plain bread flour
- ● 1 tbsp unsalted butter, softened
- ● 1 tbsp sugar
- ● 1 tsp instant dry yeast
- ● 1 tsp salt
- ● ½ cup lukewarm water

Directions:
1. Add the ingredients into the bread machine as per the order of the ingredients listed above or follow your bread machine's instruction manual.
2. Select the dough setting and press start.
3. Ten minutes into the bread machine's cycle, check on the dough to ensure that the ingredients have mixed evenly and that the dough is not too wet or dry.
4. Preheat your oven to 400 °F.
5. When ready, turn the dough out onto a floured surface and knead into a pizza or pan dish shape.
6. Top with your desired toppings and bake for 20 to 25 minutes.
Nutrition Info: (Per Serving):Calories: 536 kcal / Total fat: 7 g / Saturated fat: 4 g / Cholesterol: 15 mg / Total carbohydrates: 102 g / Dietary fiber: 4 g / Sodium: 1221 mg / Protein: 14 g

Bread Machine Pizza Dough

Servings: 1 Pizza Dough
Cooking Time: 1 Hour And 30 Minutes
Ingredients:
- Water – 1 ½ cups
- Oil – 1 ½ tbsp.
- Bread flour – 3 ¾ cups
- Sugar – 1 tbsp. plus 1 tsp.
- Salt – 1 ½ tsp.
- Active dry yeast – 1 ½ tsp.

Directions:
1. Add everything in the bread machine according to bread machine recommendations.
2. Select the Dough cycle.
3. Remove the dough when done.
4. Roll it out and bake.
Nutrition Info: (Per Serving): Calories: 40; Total Fat: 2 g; Saturated Fat: 0 g; Carbohydrates: 5 g; Cholesterol: 0 mg; Fiber: 1 g; Calcium: 14 mg; Sodium: 307 mg; Protein: 1 g

Amish Wheat Bread

Servings: 12

Cooking Time: 2 Hours 50 Minutes

Ingredients:

- 1 1/8 cups warm water
- 1 package active dry yeast
- 2 3/4 cups wheat flour
- 1/2 teaspoon salt
- 1/3 cup sugar
- 1/4 cup canola oil
- 1 large egg

Directions:

1. Add warm water, sugar and yeast to bread maker pan; let sit for 8 minutes or until it foams.
2. Add remaining ingredients to the pan.
3. Select Basic bread cycle, light crust color, and press Start.
4. Transfer to a cooling rack for 20 minutes before slicing.

Nutrition Info: Calories: 173, Sodium: 104 mg, Dietary Fiber: 0.9 g, Fat: 5.3 g, Carbs: 27.7 g, Protein: 3.7 g

Fish Bread

Servings: 10

Cooking Time: 3 Hours And 25 Minutes

Ingredients:

- Wheat bread flour – 2 ½ cups
- Bran – ½ cup
- Lukewarm water – 1 1/3 cups
- Sea salt – 1 ½ tsp.
- Sugar – 1 ½ tsp.
- Mustard oil – 1 ½ tbsp.
- Powdered milk – 2 tsp.
- Bread machine yeast – 1 ¼ tsp.
- Bell pepper – 1 cup, chopped
- Smoked fish – ¾ cup, chopped
- Onion – 1, chopped and fried

Directions:

1. Add everything in the bread machine (except onion, pepper, and fish) according to bread machine recommendations.
2. Select Basic and Medium crust.
3. Add the remaining ingredients after the beep.
4. Remove the bread when done.

5. Cool, slice, and serve.

Nutrition Info: (Per Serving): Calories: 208; Total Fat: 3.8 g; Saturated Fat: 0.5 g; Carbohydrates: 35.9 g; Cholesterol: 8 mg; Fiber: 4.2 g; Calcium: 38 mg; Sodium: 487 mg; Protein: 72 g

Bacon Breakfast Bagels

Servings: 3 Pcs

Cooking Time: 50 Minutes

Ingredients:

- Bagels
- ¾ cup (68 g) almond flour
- 1 teaspoon xanthan gum
- 1 large egg
- 1 ½ cups grated mozzarella
- 2 tablespoons cream cheese
- Toppings
- 1 tablespoon butter, melted
- Sesame seeds to taste
- Fillings
- 2 tablespoons pesto
- 2 tablespoons cream cheese
- 1 cup arugula leaves
- 6 slices grilled streaky bacon

Directions:

1. Preheat oven to 390ºF.
2. In a bowl mix together the almond flour and xanthan gum. Then add the egg and mix together until well combined. Set aside. It will look like a doughy ball.
3. In a pot over a medium-low heat slowly melt the cream cheese and mozzarella together and remove from heat once melted. This can be done in the microwave as well.
4. Add your melted cheese mix to the almond flour mix and knead until well combined. The Mozzarella mix will stick together in a bit of a ball but don't worry, persist with it. It will all combine well eventually. It's important to get the Xanthan gum incorporated through the cheese mix. Suppose the dough gets too tough to work, place in microwave for 10-20 seconds to warm and repeat until you have something that resembles a dough.
5. Split your dough into 3 pieces and roll into round logs. If you have a donut pan place your logs into the pan. If not, make circles with each log and

join together and place on a baking tray. Try to make sure you have nice little circles. The other way to do this is to make a ball and flatten slightly on the baking tray and cut a circle out of the middle if you have a small cookie cutter.

6. Melt your butter and brush over the top of your bagels and sprinkle sesame seeds or your topping of choice. The butter should help the seeds stick. Garlic and onion powder or cheese make nice additions if you have them for savory bagels.

7. Place bagels in the oven for about 18 minutes. Keep an eye on them. The tops should go golden brown.

8. Take the bagels out of the oven and allow to cool.

9. If you like your bagels toasted, cut them in half lengthwise and place back in the oven until slightly golden and toasty.

10. Spread bagel with cream cheese, cover in pesto, add a few arugula leaves and top with your crispy bacon (or your filling of choice.)

Nutrition Info: Calories: 605.67 Cal;Fats: 50.29g;Carbohydrates: 5.76g;Protein: 30.13g

Challah

Servings: 12
Cooking Time: 1 Hour 40 Minutes
Ingredients:
- 1/2 cup warm water
- 1 package active dry yeast
- 1 tablespoon sugar
- 3 tablespoons butter, softened
- 1/2 teaspoon kosher salt
- 2 to 2 1/2 cups kosher all-purpose flour
- 2 eggs
- 1 egg yolk
- 1 teaspoon water

Directions:
1. Add sugar and salt to bread maker pan.
2. Add butter, eggs, then water.
3. Add flour and yeast.
4. Select Dough cycle and press Start.
5. Transfer dough to a large mixing bowl sprayed with non-stick cooking spray. Spray dough with non-stick cooking spray and cover. Let rise in a warm place until doubled in size; about 45 minutes.

6. Punch dough down. Remove dough to lightly floured surface; pat dough and shape into a 10-by-6-inch rectangle.

7. Divide into 3 equal strips with a pizza cutter. Braid strips and place into a 9-by-5-inch loaf pan sprayed with non-stick cooking spray. Cover and let rise in warm place for about 30 to 45 minutes.

8. Beat egg yolk with 1 teaspoon water and baste loaf.

9. Bake at 375°F for 25 to 30 minutes, or until golden.

10. Let cool on a rack for 5 minutes before removing from loaf pan and serve.

Nutrition Info: Calories: 64, Sodium: 129 mg, Dietary Fiber: 0.3 g, Fat: 4 g, Carbs: 5.2 g, Protein: 1.9 g.

Fluffy Paleo Bread

Servings: 15 Slices
Cooking Time: 40 Minutes
Ingredients:
- One ¼ cup almond flour
- Five eggs
- 1 tsp. lemon juice
- 1/3 cup avocado oil
- One dash black pepper
- ½ tsp. sea salt
- 3 to 4 tbsp. tapioca flour
- 1 to 2 tsp. Poppyseed
- ¼ cup ground flaxseed
- ½ tsp. baking soda
- Top with:
- Poppy seeds
- Pumpkin seeds

Directions:
1. Preheat the oven to 350F.
2. Line a baking pan with parchment paper and set aside.
3. In a bowl, add eggs, avocado oil, and lemon juice and whisk until combined.
4. In another bowl, add tapioca flour, almond flour, baking soda, flaxseed, black pepper, and poppy seed. Mix.
5. Add the lemon juice mixture into the flour mixture and mix well.

6. Add the batter into the prepared loaf pan and top with extra pumpkin seeds and poppy seeds.

7. Cover loaf pan and transfer into the prepared oven, and bake for 20 minutes. Remove cover and bake until an inserted knife comes out clean after about 15 to 20 minutes.

8. Remove from oven and cool.

9. Slice and serve.

Nutrition Info: Calories: 149 Cal;Fat: 12.9 g;Carbohydrates: 4.4 g

Paleo Coconut Bread

Servings: 10 Pcs
Cooking Time: 50 Minutes
Ingredients:

- ½ cup coconut flour
- ¼ cup almond milk (unsweetened)
- ¼ cup coconut oil (melted)
- 6 eggs
- ¼ tsp. baking soda
- ¼ tsp. salt

Directions:

1. Preheat the oven to 350F.

2. Prepare a (8 x 4) bread pan with parchment paper.

3. In a bowl, combine salt, baking soda, and coconut flour.

4. Combine the oil, milk, and eggs in another bowl.

5. Gradually add the wet ingredients into the dry ingredients and mix well.

6. Pour the mixture into the prepared pan.

7. Bake for 40 to 50 minutes.

8. Cool, slice, and serve.

Nutrition Info: Calories: 108;Fat: 8.7g;Carb: 3.4g;Protein: 4.2g

Low-carb Bagel

Servings: 12 Pcs
Cooking Time: 25 Minutes
Ingredients:

- 1 cup protein powder, unflavored
- 1/3 cup coconut flour
- 1 tsp. baking powder
- ½ tsp. sea salt
- ¼ cup ground flaxseed

- 1/3 cup sour cream
- 12 eggs
- Seasoning topping:
- 1 tsp. dried parsley
- 1 tsp. dried oregano
- 1 tsp. Dried minced onion
- ½ tsp. Garlic powder
- ½ tsp. Dried basil
- ½ tsp. sea salt

Directions:

1. Preheat the oven to 350F.

2. In a mixer, blend sour cream and eggs until well combined.

3. Whisk together the flaxseed, salt, baking powder, protein powder, and coconut flour in a bowl.

4. Mix the dry ingredients until it becomes wet ingredients. Make sure it is well blended.

5. Whisk the topping seasoning together in a small bowl. Set aside.

6. Grease 2 donut pans that can contain six donuts each.

7. Sprinkle pan with about 1 tsp. Topping seasoning and evenly pour batter into each.

8. Sprinkle the top of each bagel evenly with the rest of the seasoning mixture.

9. Bake in the oven for 25 minutes, or until golden brown.

Nutrition Info: Calories: 134;Fat: 6.8g;Carb: 4.2g;Protein: 12.1g

Brazilian Cornbread

Servings: 12
Cooking Time: 3 Hours And 25 Minutes
Ingredients:

- Milk – 1 cup
- Water – ¼ cup
- Egg – 1
- Margarine – 3 tbsp.
- Sugar – 6 tbsp.
- Salt 1 ½ tsp.
- Yellow corn flour – 1 ½ cups
- Bread flour – 2 ½ cups
- Anise seed – 1 tsp.
- Active dry yeast – 2 ½ tsp.

Directions:

1. Add everything in the bread machine according to bread machine recommendations.
2. Select White bread and press Start.
3. Remove bread when done.
4. Cool, slice, and serve.

Nutrition Info: (Per Serving): Calories: 219.5; Total Fat: 4.9 g; Saturated Fat: 1.2 g; Carbohydrates: 38.8 g; Cholesterol: 20.5 mg; Fiber: 2.9 g; Calcium: 57 mg; Sodium: 341.5 mg; Protein: 5.3 g

Chunky Chocolate Loaf

Servings: 1 Loaf
Cooking Time: 1 Hour And 30 Minutes
Ingredients:

- ½ cup coconut flour
- ¼ cup almond flour
- ¼ cup protein powder, unsweetened
- ½ cup no-calorie sweetener of your choice
- ¼ cup dark chocolate chunks, 70% cocoa solids
- ¼ cup dark cocoa powder
- One teaspoon baking soda
- ½ teaspoon salt
- Six eggs
- ½ cup of coconut oil

Directions:
1. Put all wet ingredients first, then the dry ingredients into the bread pan.
2. Select the "Quick" or "Cake" setting of your bread machine.
3. Allow all cycles to be finished.
4. Remove the pan from the machine.
5. Wait for 10 minutes before taking out the loaf from the pan.
6. Let the loaf cool down completely before slicing it.

Nutrition Info: Calories: 206;Carbohydrates: 6g;Fat: 17g;Protein: 6g

Multigrain Sandwich Loaf

Servings: 1 Pound Loaf
Cooking Time: 3 Hours
Ingredients:

- Milk, warmed :½ cup
- Unsalted butter :2 tbsp
- Plain bread flour :1 ½ cups

- Multigrain cereal :½ cup
- Granulated brown sugar :¼ cup
- Salt :¾ tsp
- Bread machine yeast :¾ tsp

Directions:
1. Add the ingredients into the bread machine as per the order of the ingredients listed above or follow your bread machine's instruction manual.
2. Select the basic setting and medium crust function.
3. When ready, turn the bread out onto a drying rack and allow it to cool, then serve.

Nutrition Info: (Per Serving):Calories: 194 kcal / Total fat: 4.8 g / Saturated fat: 2.7 g / Cholesterol: 12 mg / Total carbohydrates: 33.1 g / Dietary fiber: 1.4 g / Sodium: 335 mg / Protein: 4.6 g

Oatmeal Bread

Servings: 1 Loaf (12 Slices)
Cooking Time: 3 Hours
Ingredients:

- 1½ teaspoon active dry yeast
- 2 cups (350 g) white bread flour, sifted
- ½ cup (100 g) oatmeal flour
- One teaspoon salt
- Two tablespoons liquid honey (can be replaced with sugar)
- ½ cup (150 ml) yogurt
- One tablespoon butter, melted
- ¾ cup (200 ml) lukewarm water (80 degrees F)
- Two tablespoons oatmeal flakes

Directions:
1. Prepare all of the ingredients for your bread and measuring means (a cup, a spoon, kitchen scales).
2. Carefully measure the ingredients into the pan.
3. Place all of the ingredients into a bread bucket in the right order and follow your bread machine's manual.
4. Close the cover.
5. Select the program of your bread machine to BASIC and choose the crust colour to MEDIUM.
6. Press START.
7. After the kneading lubricate the loaf's surface water or egg yolk and sprinkle with oat flakes.
8. Wait until the program completes.

9. When done, take the bucket out and let it cool for 5-10 minutes.

10. Shake the loaf from the pan and let cool for 30 minutes on a cooling rack.

11. Slice, serve and enjoy the taste of fragrant homemade bread.

Nutrition Info: Calories 176;Total Fat 2.3g;Saturated Fat 1.2g;Sodium 313mg;Total Carbohydrate 32.9g;Dietary Fiber 1.6g;Total Sugars 5.5g;Protein 5.5g

Whole Wheat Bread

Servings: 1 Pound Loaf

Cooking Time: 3 Hours

Ingredients:

- Lukewarm whole milk :½ cup
- Unsalted butter, diced :2 tbsp
- Whole wheat flour :1 cup
- Plain bread flour :1 cup
- Brown sugar :2 ½ tbsp
- Salt :¾ tsp
- Bread machine yeast :¾ tsp

Directions:

1. Add the ingredients into the bread machine as per the order of the ingredients listed above or follow your bread machine's instruction manual.

2. Select the whole wheat setting and medium crust function.

3. When ready, turn the bread out onto a drying rack and allow it to cool, then serve.

Nutrition Info: (Per Serving):Calories: 131.6 kcal / Total fat: 3.2 g / Saturated fat: 1.8 g / Cholesterol: 8 mg / Total carbohydrates: 22.9 g / Dietary fiber: 2.1 g / Sodium: 139.3 mg / Protein: 3.9 g

Ciabatta

Servings: 1 Pound Loaf

Cooking Time: 30 Minutes

Ingredients:

- Lukewarm water :¾ cup
- Extra-virgin olive oil :½ tbsp
- White all-purpose flour :1 ½ cups
- Salt :¾ tsp
- Sugar :½ tsp
- Bread machine yeast :¾ tsp

Directions:

1. Add the ingredients into the bread machine as per the order of the ingredients listed above or follow your bread machine's instruction manual.

2. Select the dough cycle.

3. When the dough is ready, place it onto a floured surface. Cover the dough with a ceramic or glass dish and allow it to rest for ten minutes.

4. Shape the dough an oval shape. Split into two oval shapes when doubling up on the recipe.

5. Place onto a greased baking tray, cover with a cloth and allow to rest for a further 30 minutes or until it has doubled in size. Allow the dough to rest in a dry, warm area of your kitchen.

6. Preheat your oven to 425 °F.

7. Using the bottom end of a wooden spoon make small indents on the top of each loaf. Drive the spoon down into the dough until it touches the baking tray. Then place into the oven and bake for 30 minutes.

8. Sprinkle water lightly over the top of the loaves every 10 minutes while baking.

9. When ready, turn the bread out onto a drying rack and allow it to cool, then serve.

Nutrition Info: (Per Serving):Calories: 190 kcal / Total fat: 2.2 g / Saturated fat: 0.3 g / Cholesterol: 0 mg / Total carbohydrates: 36.6 g / Dietary fiber: 1.4 g / Sodium: 441 mg / Protein: 5.1 g

Mexican Sweet Bread

Servings: 12

Cooking Time: 3 Hours

Ingredients:

- 1 cup whole milk
- 1/4 cup butter
- 1 egg
- 1/4 cup sugar
- 1 teaspoon salt
- 3 cups bread flour
- 1 1/2 teaspoons yeast

Directions:

1. Add wet ingredients to bread maker pan.

2. Add dry ingredients, except yeast.

3. Make a well in the center of the dry ingredients and add the yeast.

4. Set to Sweet Bread cycle, light crust color, and press Start.

5. Remove to a cooling rack for 15 minutes before serving.
Nutrition Info: Calories: 182, Sodium: 235 mg, Dietary Fiber: 1 g, Fat: 5.2 g, Carbs: 29.2 g, Protein: 4.6 g

Sweet Ho Yin

Servings: 15
Cooking Time: 1 Hour And 20 Minutes
Ingredients:
- Lukewarm water – 1 ¼ cups
- White bread flour – 3 cups
- Brown sugar – ¼ cup
- Salt – 1 ½ tsp.
- Butter – 1 tbsp.
- Chinese five-spice powder – 1 ½ tsp.
- Cashews – 1/3 cup, chopped
- Orange extract – 1 ½ tsp.
- Active dry yeast – 2 tsp.

Directions:
1. Combine everything in the bread machine according to bread machine recommendations.
2. Use the Regular or Rapid bake cycle.
3. Remove the bread when done.
4. Cool, slice, and serve.
Nutrition Info: (Per Serving): Calories: 128; Total Fat: 2.5 g; Saturated Fat: 0.8 g; Carbohydrates: 22.7 g; Cholesterol: 2 mg; Fiber: 1 g; Calcium: 8 mg; Sodium: 241 mg; Protein: 3.3 g

Keto Pumpkin Bread

Servings: 1 Loaf
Cooking Time: 1 Hour And 30 Minutes
Ingredients:
- 1 ½ cup almond flour
- ½ cup coconut flour
- 2/3 cup no-calorie sweetener of your choice
- ½ cup butter softened
- One teaspoon cinnamon
- ½ teaspoon nutmeg
- ½ teaspoon salt
- ¼ teaspoon ginger, grated
- 1/8 teaspoon ground cloves
- Four eggs
- ¾ cup pumpkin puree
- Four teaspoons baking powder
- One teaspoon vanilla extract

Directions:
1. Add the wet ingredients followed by dry ingredients into the bread pan.
2. Use the "Quick" or "Cake" mode of the bread machine.
3. Wait until the cycles are done.
4. Remove the pan from the machine, but take out the bread from the pan for 10 mins.
5. Let the bread cool down first before slicing it completely.
Nutrition Info: Calories: 242;Carbohydrates: 11g;Fat: 20g;Protein: 7g

Walnut Bread

Servings: 1 Loaf (20 Slices)
Cooking Time: 2 Hours
Ingredients:
- 4 cups (500 g) wheat flour, sifted
- ½ cup (130 ml) lukewarm water (80 degrees F)
- ½ cup (120 ml) lukewarm milk (80 degrees F)
- Two whole eggs
- ½ cup walnuts, fried and chopped
- One tablespoon walnut oil
- One tablespoon brown sugar
- One teaspoon salt
- One teaspoon active dry yeast

Directions:
1. Prepare all of the ingredients for your bread and measuring means (a cup, a spoon, kitchen scales).
2. Carefully measure the ingredients into the pan.
3. Place all of the ingredients into the bread bucket in the right order. Follow your manual bread machine.
4. Close the cover.
5. Select your bread machine's program to FRENCH BREAD and choose the crust colour to MEDIUM.
6. Press START.
7. Wait until the program completes.
8. When done, take the bucket out and let it cool for 5-10 minutes.
9. Shake the loaf from the pan and let cool for 30 minutes on a cooling rack.

10. Slice, serve and enjoy the taste of fragrant homemade bread.

Nutrition Info: Calories 257;Total Fat 6.7g;Saturated Fat 1g;Cholesterol 34g;Sodium 252mg;Total Carbohydrate 40.8g;Total Sugars 2g;Protein 8.3g

Butter Bread

Servings: 1 Pound Loaf
Cooking Time: 3 Hours And 35 Minutes
Ingredients:
- Egg :1
- Lukewarm whole milk :1 ¼ cup
- Unsalted butter, diced :½ cup
- Plain bread flour :2 cups
- Salt :1 pinch
- Sugar :1 pinch
- Instant dry yeast :2 tsp

Directions:
1. Add the ingredients into the bread machine as per the order of the ingredients listed above or follow your bread machine's instruction manual.
2. Select the French setting and medium crust function.
3. When ready, turn the bread out onto a drying rack and allow it to cool, then serve.

Nutrition Info: (Per Serving):Calories: 262.2 kcal / Total fat: 13.5 g / Saturated fat: 8.2 g / Cholesterol: 58.6 mg / Total carbohydrates 29.8 g / Dietary fiber: 1.3 g / Sodium: 45.3 mg / Protein: 5.9 g

Pita Bread

Servings: 8 Pcs
Cooking Time: 20 Minutes
Ingredients:
- 3 cups of all-purpose flour
- 1 1/8 cups warm water
- One tablespoon of vegetable oil
- One teaspoon salt
- 1 ½ teaspoon active dry yeast
- One active teaspoon white sugar

Directions:
1. Place all the ingredients in your bread pan.
2. Select the dough setting. Hit the start button.
3. The machine beeps after the dough rises adequately.
4. Turn the dough on a floured surface.
5. Roll and stretch the dough gently into a 12-inch rope.
6. Cut into eight pieces with a knife.
7. Now roll each piece into a ball. It should be smooth.
8. Roll each ball into a 7-inch circle. Keep covered with a towel on a floured top for 30 minutes for the pita to rise. It should get puffy slightly.
9. Preheat your oven to 260 degrees C.
10. Keep the pitas on your wire cake rack. Transfer to the oven rack directly.
11. Bake the pitas for 5 minutes. They should be puffed. The top should start to brown.
12. Take out from the oven. Keep the pitas immediately in a sealed paper bag. You can also cover using a damp kitchen towel.
13. Split the top edge or cut into half once the pitas are soft. You can also have the whole pitas if you want.

Nutrition Info: Calories 191;Carbohydrates: 37g;Total Fat 3g;Cholesterol 0mg;Protein 5g;Fiber 1g;Sugar 1g;Sodium 293mg;Potassium 66mg

Simple Dark Rye Bread

Servings: 1 Loaf (8 Slices)
Cooking Time: 2 Hours
Ingredients:
- 2/3 cup lukewarm water (80 degrees F)
- One tablespoon melted butter cooled
- ¼ cup molasses
- ¼ teaspoon salt
- One tablespoon unsweetened cocoa powder
- ½ cup rye flour
- pinch of ground nutmeg
- 1¼ cups white wheat flour sifted
- 1 1/8 teaspoons active dry yeast

Directions:
1. Prepare all of the ingredients for your bread and measuring means (a cup, a spoon, kitchen scales).
2. Carefully measure the ingredients into the pan.
3. Place all of the ingredients into the bread bucket in the right order and follow your bread machine's manual.
4. Close the cover.

5. Select the program of your bread machine to BASIC and choose the crust colour to MEDIUM.

6. Wait until the program completes.

7. When done, take the bucket out and let it cool for 5-10 minutes.

8. Shake the loaf from the pan and let cool for 30 minutes on a cooling rack.

9. Slice, serve and enjoy the taste of fragrant homemade bread.

Nutrition Info: Calories 151;Total Fat 2.1g;Saturated Fat 1g;Cholesterol 4g;Sodium 88mg;Total Carbohydrate 29.4g;Dietary Fiber 2.7g;Total Sugars 5.9g;Protein 4.2g

European Black Bread

Servings: 1 Loaf
Cooking Time: 1 Hour And 5 Minutes
Ingredients:

- ¾ teaspoon cider vinegar
- 1 cup of water
- ½ cup rye flour
- 1 ½ cups flour
- One tablespoon margarine
- ¼ cup of oat bran
- One teaspoon salt
- 1 ½ tablespoons sugar
- One teaspoon dried onion flakes
- One teaspoon caraway seed
- One teaspoon yeast
- Two tablespoons unsweetened cocoa

Directions:

1. Put everything in your bread machine.
2. Now select the basic setting.
3. Hit the start button.
4. Transfer bread to a rack for cooling once done.

Nutrition Info: Calories 114;Carbohydrates: 22 g;Total Fat 1.7 g;Cholesterol 0mg;Protein 3 g;Sugar 2 g;Sodium 247 mg

No Sugar-added Pizza Dough

Servings: 2 Pizzas
Cooking Time: 1 Hour And 30 Minutes
Ingredients:

- Warm water – 1 cup, 105ºF to 115ºF
- Oil – 2 tbsp.

- Salt – 1 tsp.
- Unbleached all-purpose flour – 3 cups
- Active dry yeast – 1 tbsp.

Directions:

1. Add everything in the bread machine according to bread machine recommendations.
2. Select the Dough setting and press Start.
3. Transfer the dough on a lightly floured work surface when done. Knead and divide in half.
4. Make 2 balls and cover with a clean towel. Allow to rise in a warm place for 40 minutes.
5. Bake.

Nutrition Info: (Per Serving): Calories: 820; Total Fat: 16.1 g; Saturated Fat: 2.3 g; Carbohydrates: 145.4 g; Cholesterol: 0 mg; Fiber: 6.3 g; Calcium: 36 mg; Sodium: 1,173 mg; Protein: 21.7 g

Syrian Bread

Servings: 8 Pcs
Cooking Time: 20 Minutes
Ingredients:

- Two tablespoons vegetable oil
- 1 cup of water
- 1 ½ teaspoons salt
- ½ teaspoon white sugar
- 1 ½ teaspoon active dry yeast
- 3 cups all-purpose flour

Directions:

1. Put everything in your bread machine pan.
2. Select the dough cycle. Hit the start button.
3. Preheat your oven to 475 degrees F.
4. Turn to dough on a lightly floured surface once done.
5. Divide it into eight equal pieces. Form them into rounds.
6. Take a damp cloth and cover the rounds with it.
7. Now roll the dough into flat thin circles. They should have a diameter of around 8 inches.
8. Cook in your preheated baking sheets until they are golden brown and puffed.

Nutrition Info: Calories 204;Carbohydrates: 36g;Total Fat 5g;Cholesterol 0mg;Protein 5g;Fiber 1g;Sugar 0g;Sodium 438mg;Potassium 66mg

Bacon And Cheese Bread

Servings: 1 Pound Loaf

Cooking Time: 3 Hours
Ingredients:
- Egg, lightly beaten :½
- Lukewarm water :½ cup
- Unsalted butter, diced :½ tbsp
- Shredded cheddar cheese :½ cup
- Bacon bits :2 tbsp
- Plain bread flour :2 cups
- Salt :½ tsp
- Sugar :1 tbsp
- Active dry yeast :1 tsp

Directions:
1. Add the ingredients into the bread machine as per the order of the ingredients listed above or follow your bread machine's instruction manual.
2. Select the basic cycle and light crust function.
3. When ready, turn the bread out onto a drying rack and allow it to cool, then serve.

Nutrition Info: (Per Serving):Calories: 171.3 kcal / Total fat: 4.6 g / Saturated fat: 2.5 g / Cholesterol: 26.9 mg / Total carbohydrates: 25.8 g / Dietary fiber: 1 g / Sodium: 283.1 mg / Protein: 6.2 g

Ethiopian Milk And Honey Bread

Servings: 1 Loaf
Cooking Time: 1 Hour And 15 Minutes
Ingredients:
- Three tablespoons honey
- 1 cup + 1 tablespoon milk
- 3 cups bread flour
- Three tablespoons melted butter
- Two teaspoons active dry yeast
- 1 ½ teaspoons salt

Directions:
1. Add everything to the pan of your bread
2. Select the white bread or basic setting and the medium crust setting.
3. Hit the start button.
4. Take out your hot loaf once it is done.
5. Keep on your wire rack for cooling.
6. Slice your bread once it is cold and serve.

Nutrition Info: Calories 129;Carbohydrates: 20 g;Total Fat 3.8 g;Cholesterol 0 mg;Protein 2.4 g;Fiber 0.6 g;Sugars 3.3 g;Sodium 78 mg

Soft Pretzels

Servings: 24 Pcs

Cooking Time: 20 Minutes
Ingredients:
- oz. cocoa butter
- ½ cup coconut butter
- ½ cup sugar-free maple syrup
- 1/3 cup heavy cream
- 3 tbsp coconut oil
- Two scoops matcha MCT powder
- 2 tsp vanilla essence

Directions:
1. Start by throwing all the ingredients into a saucepan.
2. Stir cook on low heat until butter is melted, then stir well.
3. Spread this mixture in an 8x8-inch pan lined with parchment paper.
4. Refrigerate for 3 hours, then slice into 24 pieces.

Nutrition Info: Calories 173;Total Fat 13 g;Saturated Fat 10.1 g;Cholesterol 12 mg;Sodium 67 mg;Total Carbs 7.5 g;Sugar 1.2 g;Fibre 0.6 g;Protein 3.2 g

German Rye Bread

Servings: 20
Cooking Time: 3 Hour And 48 Minutes
Ingredients:
- Buttermilk – 1 ½ cups
- Whole wheat flour – 2 ½ cups
- Rye flour – ½ cup
- Bread flour – ½ cup
- Buckwheat flour – ¼ cup
- Wheat germ – ¼ cup
- Salt - 1 tsp.
- Flax seeds – ¼ cup
- Soft butter – 1 tbsp.
- Molasses – 3 tbsp.
- Active dry yeast – 3 tsp.

Directions:
1. Add everything according to the bread machine recommendations.
2. Select Whole Grain and Dark crust.
3. Remove the bread when done.
4. Cool, slice, and serve.

Nutrition Info: (Per Serving): Calories: 151; Total Fat: 4 g; Saturated Fat: 2.3 g; Carbohydrates: 23.8 g; Cholesterol: 10 mg; Fiber: 2.4 g; Calcium: 93 mg; Sodium: 193 mg; Protein: 5.6 g

Sweet Pizza Dough

Servings: 1 Pizza
Cooking Time: 1 Hour And 30 Minutes
Ingredients:
- Dried granulated yeast – 2 tsp.
- Bread flour – 3 cups
- Salt – 1 tsp.
- Sugar – 2 tbsp.
- Oil – 2 tbsp.
- Water – 1 cup, and more if needed
- Water – 2 tbsp.

Directions:
1. Place everything in the bread machine according to bread machine recommendations.
2. Select Dough cycle and press Start.
3. When finished, remove the dough and place it in a greased bowl. Roll the dough around so it is coated with oil.
4. Cover and allow to rise for ½ hour in a warm place. Knead the dough.
5. Shake and bake.

Nutrition Info: (Per Serving): Calories: 1727.2; Total Fat: 31.3 g; Saturated Fat: 4.4 g; Carbohydrates: 314.7 g; Cholesterol: 0 mg; Fiber: 12.3 g; Calcium: 144 mg; Sodium: 2,345.8 mg; Protein: 42 g

Dinner Rolls

Servings: 15 Rolls
Cooking Time: 2 Hours And 35 Minutes
Ingredients:
- 1 egg
- 1 cup water
- 3 ¼ cups plain bread flour
- ¼ cup sugar
- 1 tsp salt
- 3 tsp active dry yeast
- 2 tbsp unsalted butter, softened

Directions:
1. Add the ingredients into the bread machine as per the order of the ingredients listed above or follow your bread machine's instruction manual. Do not add the softened butter in.
2. Select the dough setting.
3. Transfer the dough onto a floured surface and allow to rest for 10 minutes. Then split the dough evenly into 15 balls.

4. On a greased baking tray, place the dough balls 2" apart. Allow the rolls to rest in a warm area for 30 minutes or until they have doubled in size.
5. Preheat your oven to 375 °F and bake the rolls for 15 minutes or until they have turned a honeyed color.
6. Brush the tops of the rolls with the softened butter, then serve.

Nutrition Info: (Per Serving):Calories: 135 kcal / Total fat: 2 g / Saturated fat: 0 g / Cholesterol: 15 mg / Total carbohydrates: 26 g / Dietary fiber: 1 g / Sodium: 170 mg / Protein: 4 g

No-bake Butter Cookies

Servings: 8 Pcs
Cooking Time: 0 Minutes
Ingredients:
- ½ cup almond flour
- 1½ tbsp butter
- 1 tbsp Swerve
- ½ tsp vanilla extract
- 1 pinch salt

Directions:
1. Mix all the ingredients in a bowl to prepare the cookie batter.
2. Spoon out the batter onto a cookie sheet positioned on a baking tray.
3. Put the tray in the refrigerator and refrigerate for about 1 hour 10 minutes.
4. Serve the cookies.

Nutrition Info: Calories: 125 Cal;Fat: 3.2 g;Cholesterol: 11 mg;Sodium: 75 mg;Carbohydrates: 3,6 g

Fiji Sweet Potato Bread

Servings: 1 Loaf
Cooking Time: 1 Hour And 10minutes
Ingredients:
- One teaspoon vanilla extract
- ½ cup of warm water
- 4 cups flour
- 1 cup sweet mashed potatoes
- Two tablespoons softened butter
- ½ teaspoon cinnamon
- 1 ½ teaspoons salt
- 1/3 cup brown sugar
- Two tablespoons powdered milk

- Two teaspoons yeast

Directions:
1. Add everything in the pan of your bread.
2. Select the white bread and the crust you want.
3. Hit the start button.
4. Set aside on wire racks for cooling before slicing.

Nutrition Info: Calories: 168 Cal;Carbohydrates: 28 g;Fat: 5g;Cholesterol: 0 mg;Protein: 4 g;Fiber: 1g;Sugat 3 g;Sodium: 292 mg

White Chocolate Bread

Servings: 1 Loaf
Cooking Time: 2 Hours And 55 Minutes
Ingredients:
- ¼ cup warm water
- 1 cup warm milk
- 1 egg
- ¼ cup butter, softened
- 3 cups bread flour
- 2 tablespoons brown sugar
- 2 tablespoons white sugar
- 1 teaspoon salt
- 1 teaspoon ground cinnamon
- 1 (.25 ounce) package active dry yeast
- 1 cup white chocolate chips

Directions:
1. Place all ingredients (except the white chocolate chips) in the pan of the bread machine in the order recommended by the manufacturer.
2. Select cycle; press Start.
3. If your machine has a Fruit setting, add the white chocolate chips at the signal, otherwise you can do it about 5 minutes before the kneading cycle has finished.

Nutrition Info: Calories 277 ;Protein 6.6g;Carbohydrates 39g;Fat: 10.5g

Finnish Pulla

Servings: 1 Loaf
Cooking Time: 30 Minutes
Ingredients:
- 1 cup milk
- 1/4 cup water, lukewarm
- 3 eggs, 1 egg reserved for glaze
- 4 1/2 cups all purpose flour
- 1/2 cup sugar
- 1 teaspoon salt

- 1 tablespoon ground cardamom
- 1 tablespoon yeast
- 1/4 cup butter, cut into 4 chunks
- 1-2 tablespoons pearl sugar for topping loaves

Directions:
1. Place the milk, water, and 2 lightly beaten eggs in bread machine pan.
2. Add flour, sugar, salt, cardamom in the pan, then top it with yeast and butter. Program the bread machine to dough setting.
3. Remove the dough from the bread machine pan and place on a lightly floured surface. Divide the dough into 3 equal pieces. Roll each piece of dough into 10-14 inch strand and braid. Pinch and tuck the ends under and place on greased or parchment covered baking sheet. Lightly cover it with a clean kitchen towel and let it rise for about 30-45 minutes.
4. Preheat the oven to 325 degrees. Beat the remaining egg and gently brush the loaf on top and on the sides with pastry brush. Sprinkle with pearl sugar. Bake for 20 to 25 minutes until it becomes light golden brown. Cool on wire rack, then slice to serve.

Nutrition Information:
- ;Total Fat 4.5g;Saturated fat 2.5g;Cholesterol 35mg;Sodium 140mg;Carbohydrates 26g;Net carbs 25g;Sugar 5g;Fiber 1g;Protein 4g

Rice Wheat Bread

Servings: 1 Loaf (22 Slices)
Cooking Time: 1 Hour And 30 Minutes
Ingredients:
- 4½ cups (580 g) wheat bread flour
- 1 cup (200 g) rice, cooked
- One whole egg
- Two tablespoons soy sauce
- Two teaspoons active dried yeast
- Two tablespoons melted butter
- One tablespoon brown sugar
- Two teaspoons kosher salt

Directions:
1. Prepare all of the ingredients for your bread and measuring means (a cup, a spoon, kitchen scales).
2. Carefully measure the ingredients into the pan.
3. Place all of the ingredients into a bucket in the right order. Follow your manual for the bread machine.

4. Close the cover.
5. Select the program of your bread machine to BASIC and choose the crust colour to MEDIUM.
6. Press START.
7. Wait until the program completes.
8. When done, take the bucket out and let it cool for 5-10 minutes.
9. Shake the loaf from the pan and let cool for 30 minutes on a cooling rack.
10. Slice, serve and enjoy the taste of fragrant homemade bread.

Nutrition Info: Calories 321;Total Fat 4.2g;Saturated Fat 2.1g;Cholesterol 28g;Sodium 837mg;Total Carbohydrate 60.4g;Dietary Fiber 2.2g;Total Sugars 1.4g;Protein 9.1g

Portuguese Sweet Bread

Servings: 1 Loaf
Cooking Time: 1 Hour And 5 Minutes
Ingredients:
- One egg beaten
- 1 cup milk
- 1/3 cup sugar
- Two tablespoons margarine
- 3 cups bread flour
- ¾ teaspoon salt
- 2 ½ teaspoons active dry yeast

Directions:
1. Place everything into your bread machine.
2. Select the sweet bread setting. Hit the start button.

3. Transfer the loaves to a rack for cooling once done.

Nutrition Info: Calories 139;Carbohydrates: 24 g;Total Fat 8.3 g;Cholesterol 14 mg;Protein 3 g;Fiber 0g;Sugar 4 g;Sodium 147 mg

French Ham Bread

Servings: 10
Cooking Time: 3 Hours And 27 Minutes
Ingredients:
- Wheat bread flour – 3 1/3 cups
- Ham – 1 cup, chopped
- Milk powder – ½ cup
- Sugar – 1 ½ tbsp.
- Fresh yeast – 1 tsp.
- Kosher salt – 1 tsp.
- Parmesan cheese – 2 tbsp., grated
- Lukewarm water – 1 1/3 cups
- Oil – 2 tbsp.

Directions:
1. Add everything (except for the ham) in the bread machine according to bread machine recommendations.
2. Select French bread and Medium crust.
3. Add ham after the beep.
4. Remove the bread when done.
5. Cool, slice, and serve.

Nutrition Info: (Per Serving): Calories: 287; Total Fat: 5.5 g; Saturated Fat: 1.1 g; Carbohydrates: 47.2 g; Cholesterol: 11 mg; Fiber: 1.7 g; Calcium: 65 mg; Sodium: 557 mg; Protein: 11.4 g

BASIC BREAD

Anadama Bread

Servings: 2 Loaves
Cooking Time: 45 Minutes
Ingredients:
- 1/2 cup sunflower seeds
- Two teaspoons bread machine yeast
- 4 1/2 cups bread flour
- 3/4 cup yellow cornmeal
- Two tablespoons unsalted butter, cubed
- 1 1/2 teaspoon salt
- 1/4 cup dry skim milk powder
- 1/4 cup molasses
- 1 1/2 cups water, with a temperature of 80 to 90 degrees F (26 to 32 degrees C)

Directions:
1. Put all the pan's ingredients, except the sunflower seeds, in this order: water, molasses, milk, salt, butter, cornmeal, flour, and yeast.
2. Put the pan in the machine and cover the lid.
3. Put the sunflower seeds in the fruit and nut dispenser.
4. Turn the machine on and choose the basic setting and your desired colour of the crust—press start.

Nutrition Info: Calories: 130 calories;Total Carbohydrate: 25 g ;Total Fat: 2 g ;Protein: 3 g

100 Percent Whole-wheat Bread

Servings: 1 Loaf
Cooking Time: 10 Minutes Or Less
Ingredients:
- 12 slice bread (1½ pound)
- 1⅛ cups water, at 80°F to 90°F
- 2¼ tablespoons melted butter, cooled
- 2¼ tablespoons honey
- 1⅛ teaspoons salt
- 3 cups whole-wheat bread flour
- 2 teaspoons sugar
- 2 tablespoons skim milk powder
- ¾ teaspoon salt
- 1½ teaspoons bread machine or instant yeast

Directions:
1. Preparing the Ingredients.

2. Choose the size of bread to prepare. Measure and add the ingredients to the pan in the order as indicated in the ingredient listing. Place the pan in the bread machine and close the lid.
3. Select the Bake cycle
4. Turn on the bread maker. Select the Wheat/ Whole setting, then select the dough size and crust color. Press start to start the cycle. When this is done, and the bread is baked, remove the pan from the machine. Let stand a few minutes.
5. Remove the bread from the pan and leave it on a wire rack to cool for at least 10 minutes. Slice and serve.

Coconut Flour Bread

Servings: 12 Pcs
Cooking Time: 15 Minutes
Ingredients:
- 6 eggs
- 1/2 cup coconut flour
- 2 tbsp psyllium husk
- 1/4 cup olive oil
- 1 1/2 tsp salt
- 1 tbsp xanthan gum
- 1 tbsp baking powder
- 2 1/4 tsp yeast

Directions:
1. Use a small bowl to combine all of the dry ingredients except for the yeast.
2. In the bread machine pan, add all the wet ingredients.
3. Add all of your dry ingredients from the small mixing bowl to the bread machine pan. Top with the yeast.
4. Set the machine to the basic setting.
5. When the bread is finished, remove the bread machine pan from the bread machine.
6. Let cool slightly before transferring to a cooling rack.
7. It can be stored for four days on the counter and up to 3 months in the freezer.

Nutrition Info: Calories: 174 ;Carbohydrates: 4g ;Protein: 7g ;Fat: 15g

Zero-fat Carrot And Pinapple Loaf

Servings: 1 Loaf
Cooking Time: 1 Hour And 30 Minutes
Ingredients:

- 2 ½ cups all-purpose flour
- ¾ cup of sugar
- ½ cup pineapples, crushed
- ½ cup carrots, grated
- ½ cup raisins
- Two teaspoons baking powder
- ½ teaspoon ground cinnamon
- ½ teaspoon salt
- ¼ teaspoon allspice
- ¼ teaspoon nutmeg
- ½ cup applesauce
- One tablespoon molasses

Directions:

1. Put first the wet ingredients into the bread pan before the dry ingredients.
2. Press the "Quick" or "Cake" mode of your bread machine.
3. Allow the machine to complete all cycles.
4. Take out the pan from the machine, but wait for another 10 minutes before transferring the bread into a wire rack.
5. Cooldown the bread before slicing.

Nutrition Info: Calories: 70;Carbohydrates: 16g;Fat: 0g;Protein: 1g

Classic White Bread I

Servings: 1 Loaf
Cooking Time: 10 Minutes
Ingredients:

- 16 slice bread (2 pounds)
- 1½ cups lukewarm water
- 1 tablespoon + 1 teaspoon olive oil
- 1½ teaspoons sugar
- 1 teaspoon table salt
- ¼ teaspoon baking soda
- 2½ cups all-purpose flour
- 1 cup white bread flour
- 2½ teaspoons bread machine yeast

Directions:

1. Preparing the Ingredients

2. Choose the size of bread to prepare. Measure and add the ingredients to the pan in the order as indicated in the ingredient listing. Place the pan in the bread machine and close the lid.
3. Select the Bake cycle
4. Close the lid, Turn on the bread maker. Select the White / Basic setting, then select the dough size and crust color. Press start to start the cycle.
5. When this is done, and the bread is baked, remove the pan from the machine. Let stand a few minutes.
6. Remove the bread from the pan and leave it on a wire rack to cool for at least 10 minutes.
7. After this time, proceed to cut it

Whole Wheat Breakfast Bread

Servings: 14 Slices
Cooking Time: 3 H. 5 Min.
Ingredients:

- 3 cups white whole wheat flour
- ½ tsp salt
- 1 cup water
- ½ cup coconut oil, liquified
- 4 Tbsp honey
- 2½ tsp active dry yeast

Directions:

1. Add each ingredient to the bread machine in the order and at the temperature recommended by your bread machine manufacturer.
2. Close the lid, select the basic bread, medium crust setting on your bread machine and press start.
3. When the bread machine has finished baking, remove the bread and put it on a cooling rack.

Pumpkin Raisin Bread

Servings: 1 Loaf
Cooking Time: 1 Hour And 30 Minutes
Ingredients:

- ½ cup all-purpose flour
- ½ cup whole-wheat flour
- ½ cup pumpkin, mashed
- ½ cup raisins
- ¼ cup brown sugar
- Two tablespoons baking powder
- One teaspoon salt

- One teaspoon pumpkin pie spice
- ¼ teaspoon baking soda
- ¾ cup apple juice
- ¼ cup of vegetable oil
- Three tablespoons aquafaba

Directions:

1. Place all ingredients in the bread pan in this order: apple juice, pumpkin, oil, aquafaba, flour, sugar, baking powder, baking soda, salt, pumpkin pie spice, and raisins.
2. Select the "Quick" or "Cake" mode of your bread machine.
3. Let the machine finish all cycles.
4. Remove the pan from the machine.
5. After 10 minutes, transfer the bread to a wire rack.
6. Slice the bread only when it has completely cooled down.

Nutrition Info: Calories: 70;Carbohydrates: 12g;Fat: 2g;Protein: 1g

Honey Whole-wheat Sandwich Bread

Servings: 14 Slices
Cooking Time: 3 H.

Ingredients:

- 4¼ cups whole-wheat flour
- ½ tsp salt
- 1½ cups water
- ¼ cup honey
- 2 Tbsp olive oil, or melted butter
- 2¼ tsp bread machine yeast (1 packet)

Directions:

1. Add each ingredient to the bread machine in the order and at the temperature recommended by your bread machine manufacturer.
2. Close the lid, select the whole wheat, low crust setting on your bread machine and press start.
3. When the bread machine has finished baking, remove the bread and put it on a cooling rack.

Double-chocolate Zucchini Bread

Servings: 1 Loaf
Cooking Time: 10 Minutes

Ingredients:

- 225 grams grated zucchini

- 125 grams All-Purpose Flour Blend
- 50 grams all-natural unsweetened cocoa powder (not Dutch-process)
- 1 teaspoon xanthan gum
- ¾ teaspoon baking soda
- ¼ teaspoon baking powder
- ¼ teaspoon salt
- ½ teaspoon ground espresso
- 135 grams chocolate chips or nondairy alternative
- 100 grams cane sugar or granulated sugar
- 2 large eggs
- ¼ cup avocado oil or canola oil
- 60 grams vanilla Greek yogurt or nondairy alternative
- 1 teaspoon vanilla extract

Directions:

1. Preparing the Ingredients.
2. Measure and add the ingredients to the pan in the order mentioned above. Place the pan in the bread machine and close the lid.
3. Select the Bake cycle
4. Turn on the bread maker. Select the White / Basic setting, then select the dough size, select light or medium crust. Press start to start the cycle.
5. When this is done, and the bread is baked, remove the pan from the machine. Let stand a few minutes.
6. Remove the bread from the skillet and leave it on a wire rack to cool for at least 15 minutes. Store leftovers in an airtight container at room temperature for up to 5 days, or freeze to enjoy a slice whenever you desire. Let each slice thaw naturally

Anadama White Bread

Servings: 14 Slices
Cooking Time: 3 H.

Ingredients:

- 1⅛ cups water (110°F/43°C)
- ⅓ cup molasses
- 1½ Tbsp butter at room temperature
- 1 tsp salt
- ⅓ cup yellow cornmeal
- 3½ cups bread flour

- 2½ tsp bread machine yeast

Directions:

1. Add each ingredient to the bread machine in the order and at the temperature recommended by your bread machine manufacturer.

2. Close the lid, select the basic bread, low crust setting on your bread machine, and press start.

3. When the bread machine has finished baking, remove the bread and put it on a cooling rack.

Pumpernickel Bread 3

Servings: 12
Cooking Time: 3 Hours 30 Minutes
Ingredients:

- 1 1/4 cups lukewarm water
- 1/4 cup molasses
- 2 tablespoons unsweetened cocoa powder
- 1 teaspoon sea salt
- 1 cup whole wheat flour
- 1 cup rye flour
- 2 cups unbleached all-purpose flour
- 2 1/2 tablespoons vegetable oil
- 1 1/2 tablespoons packed brown sugar
- 1 tablespoon caraway seeds
- 2 1/2 teaspoons instant yeast

Directions:

1. Add all of the ingredients in the order listed above, reserving yeast.

2. Make a well in the center of the dry ingredients and add the yeast .

3. Set the bread maker on Whole Wheat cycle, select crust color, and press Start.

4. Remove and let the loaf cool for 15 minutes before slicing.

5. Note: all ingredients should be at room temperature before baking.

Nutrition Info: Calories: 263, Sodium: 160 mg, Dietary Fiber: 4.7 g, Fat: 3.5 g, Carbs: 50.6 g, Protein: 7.1 g.

Traditional Italian Bread

Servings: 1 Loaf
Cooking Time: 10 Minutes
Ingredients:

- 12 slice bread (1½ pounds)

- 1 cup water, at 80°F to 90°F
- 1½ tablespoons olive oil
- 1½ tablespoons sugar
- 1⅛ teaspoons salt
- 3 cups white bread flour
- 2⅔ cups white bread flour
- 1½ teaspoons bread machine or instant yeast

Directions:

1. Preparing the Ingredients.

2. Place the ingredients in your bread machine as recommended by the manufacturer

3. Select the Bake cycle

4. Close the lid, Turn on the bread maker. Select the White / Basic setting, then select the dough size, select light or medium crust. Press start to start the cycle.

5. When this is done, and the bread is baked, remove the pan from the machine. Let stand a few minutes.

6. Remove the bread from the skillet and leave it on a wire rack to cool for at least 10 minutes. Slice and serve.

Mustard Flavoured General Bread

Servings: 2 Loaves
Cooking Time: 40 Minutes
Ingredients:

- 1¼ cups milk
- Three tablespoons sunflower milk
- Three tablespoons sour cream
- Two tablespoons dry mustard
- One whole egg beaten
- ½ sachet sugar vanilla
- 4 cups flour
- One teaspoon dry yeast
- Two tablespoons sugar
- Two teaspoon salt

Directions:

1. Take out the bread maker's bucket and pour in milk and sunflower oil stir and then add sour cream and beaten egg.

2. Add flour, salt, sugar, mustard powder, vanilla sugar, and mix well.

3. Make a small groove in the flour and sprinkle the yeast.

4. Transfer the bucket to your bread maker and cover.

5. Set the program of your bread machine to Basic/White Bread and set crust type to Medium.

6. Press START.

7. Wait until the cycle completes.

8. Once the loaf is ready, take the bucket out and let it cool for 5 minutes.

9. Gently shake the bucket to remove the loaf.

10. Transfer to a cooling rack, slice, and serve.

Nutrition Info: Calories: 340 Cal;Fat: 10 g ;Carbohydrates:54 g ;Protein: 10 g ;Fibre: 1 g

Molasses Wheat Bread

Servings: 1 Loaf
Cooking Time: 10 Minutes Or Less
Ingredients:

- 12 slice bread (1½ pound)
- ¾ cup water, at 80°F to 90°F
- ⅓ cup milk, at 80°F
- 1 tablespoon melted butter, cooled
- 3¾ tablespoons honey
- 2 tablespoons molasses
- 2 teaspoons sugar
- 2 tablespoons skim milk powder
- ¾ teaspoon salt
- 2 teaspoons unsweetened cocoa powder
- 1¾ cups whole-wheat flour
- 1¼ cups white bread flour
- 1⅛ teaspoons bread machine yeast or instant yeast

Directions:

1. Preparing the Ingredients.

2. Choose the size of bread to prepare. Measure and add the ingredients to the pan in the order as indicated in the ingredient listing. Place the pan in the bread machine and close the lid.

3. Select the Bake cycle

4. Turn on the bread maker. Select the White / Basic setting, then select the dough size and crust color. Press start to start the cycle.

5. When this is done, and the bread is baked, remove the pan from the machine. Let stand a few minutes.

6. Remove the bread from the pan and leave it on a wire rack to cool for at least 10 minutes.

7. After this time, proceed to cut it.

Southern Cornbread

Servings: 10
Cooking Time: 1 Hour
Ingredients:

- 2 fresh eggs, at room temperature
- 1 cup milk
- 1/4 cup butter, unsalted, at room temperature
- 3/4 cup sugar
- 1 teaspoon salt
- 2 cups unbleached all-purpose flour
- 1 cup cornmeal
- 1 tablespoon baking powder

Directions:

1. Add all of the ingredients to your bread maker in the order listed.

2. Select the Quick Bread cycle, light crust color, and press Start.

3. Allow to cool for five minutes on a wire rack and serve warm.

Nutrition Info: Calories: 258, Sodium: 295 mg, Dietary Fiber: 1.6 g, Fat: 6.7 g, Carbs: 45.4 g, Protein: 5.5 g.

Italian White Bread

Servings: 14 Slices
Cooking Time: 3 H.
Ingredients:

- ¾ cup cold water
- 2 cups bread flour
- 1 Tbsp sugar
- 1 tsp salt
- 1 Tbsp olive oil
- 1 tsp active dry yeast

Directions:

1. Add each ingredient to the bread machine in the order and at the temperature recommended by your bread machine manufacturer.

2. Close the lid, select the Italian or basic bread, low crust setting on your bread machine, and press start.

3. When the bread machine has finished baking, remove the bread and put it on a cooling rack.

Homemade Wonderful Bread

Servings: 2 Loaves
Cooking Time: 15 Minutes
Ingredients:

- 2 1/2 teaspoons active dry yeast
- 1/4 cup warm water
- One tablespoon white sugar
- 4 cups all-purpose flour
- 1/4 cup dry potato flakes
- 1/4 cup dry milk powder
- Two teaspoons salt
- 1/4 cup white sugar
- Two tablespoons margarine
- 1 cup of warm water(45 degrees C)

Directions:

1. Prepare the yeast, 1/4 cup warm water and sugar to whisk and then let it sit in 15 minutes.
2. Take all ingredients together with yeast mixture to put in the pan of bread machine according to the manufacturer's recommended order. Choose basic and light crust settings.

Nutrition Info: Calories: 162 calories;Total Carbohydrate: 31.6 g ;Cholesterol: < 1 mg ;Total Fat: 1.8 g ;Protein: 4.5 g

Autumn Treasures Loaf

Servings: 1 Loaf
Cooking Time: 1 Hour And 30 Minutes
Ingredients:

- 1 cup all-purpose flour
- ½ cup dried fruit, chopped
- ¼ cup pecans, chopped
- ¼ cup of sugar
- Two tablespoons baking powder
- One teaspoon salt
- ¼ teaspoon of baking soda
- ½ teaspoon ground nutmeg
- 1 cup apple juice
- ¼ cup of vegetable oil
- Three tablespoons aquafaba
- One teaspoon of vanilla extract

Directions:

1. Add all wet ingredients first to the bread pan before the dry ingredients.

2. Turn on the bread machine with the "Quick" or "Cake" setting.
3. Wait for all cycles to be finished.
4. Remove the bread pan from the machine.
5. After 10 minutes, transfer the bread from the pan into a wire rack.
6. Slice the bread only when it has completely cooled down.

Nutrition Info: Calories: 80;Carbohydrates: 12g;Fat: 3g;Protein: 1g

Cracked Wheat Bread

Servings: 10
Cooking Time: 1 Hour 20 Minutes
Ingredients:

- 1 1/4 cup plus 1 tablespoon water
- 2 tablespoons vegetable oil
- 3 cups bread flour
- 3/4 cup cracked wheat
- 1 1/2 teaspoons salt
- 2 tablespoons sugar
- 2 1/4 teaspoons active dry yeast

Directions:

1. Bring water to a boil.
2. Place cracked wheat in small mixing bowl, pour water over it and stir.
3. Cool to 80°F.
4. Place cracked wheat mixture into pan, followed by all ingredients (except yeast) in the order listed.
5. Make a well in the center of the dry ingredients and add the yeast.
6. Select the Basic Bread cycle, medium color crust, and press Start.
7. Check dough consistency after 5 minutes of kneading. The dough should be a soft, tacky ball. If it is dry and stiff, add water one 1/2 tablespoon at a time until sticky. If it's too wet and sticky, add 1 tablespoon of flour at a time.
8. Remove bread when cycle is finished and allow to cool before serving.

Nutrition Info: Calories: 232, Sodium: 350 mg, Dietary Fiber: 3.3 g, Fat: 3.3 g, Carbs: 43.7 g, Protein: 6.3 g.

Vegan White Bread

Servings: 14 Slices
Cooking Time: 3 H.
Ingredients:
- 1⅓ cups water
- ⅓ cup plant milk (I use silk soy original)
- 1½ tsp salt
- 2 Tbsp granulated sugar
- 2 Tbsp vegetable oil
- 3½ cups all-purpose flour
- 1¾ tsp bread machine yeast

Directions:
1. Add each ingredient to the bread machine in the order and at the temperature recommended by your bread machine manufacturer.
2. Close the lid, select the basic or white bread, medium crust setting on your bread machine, and press start.
3. When the bread machine has finished baking, remove the bread and put it on a cooling rack.

Luscious White Bread

Servings: 10
Cooking Time: 2 Hours
Ingredients:
- Warm milk – 1 cup.
- Eggs – 2
- Butter – 2 ½ tbsps.
- Sugar – ¼ cup.
- Salt – ¾ tsp.
- Bread flour – 3 cups.
- Yeast – 2 ½ tsps.

Directions:
1. Add all ingredients to the bread machine pan according to the bread machine manufacturer instructions. Select basic bread setting then select light crust and start. Once loaf is done, remove the loaf pan from the machine. Allow it to cool for 10 minutes. Slice and serve.

Easy Gluten-free, Dairy-free Bread

Servings: 12
Cooking Time: 15 Minutes
Ingredients:

- 1 1/2 cups warm water
- 2 teaspoons active dry yeast
- 2 teaspoons sugar
- 2 eggs, room temperature
- 1 egg white, room temperature
- 1 1/2 tablespoons apple cider vinegar
- 4 1/2 tablespoons olive oil
- 3 1/3 cups multi-purpose gluten-free flour

Directions:
1. Preparing the Ingredients
2. Add the yeast and sugar to the warm water and stir to mix in a large mixing bowl; set aside until foamy, about 8 to 10 minutes.
3. Whisk the 2 eggs and 1 egg white together in a separate mixing bowl and add to baking pan of bread maker.
4. Add apple cider vinegar and oil to baking pan.
5. Add foamy yeast/water mixture to baking pan.
6. Add the multi-purpose gluten-free flour on top.
7. Select the Bake cycle
8. Set for Gluten-Free bread setting and Start.
9. Remove and invert pan onto a cooling rack to remove the bread from the baking pan. Allow to cool completely before slicing to serve.

Buttermilk White Bread

Servings: 1 Loaf
Cooking Time: 25 Minutes
Ingredients:
- 1 1/8 cups water
- Three teaspoon honey
- One tablespoon margarine
- 1 1/2 teaspoon salt
- 3 cups bread flour
- Two teaspoons active dry yeast
- Four teaspoons powdered buttermilk

Directions:
1. Into the bread machine's pan, place the ingredients in the order suggested by the manufacturer: select medium crust and white bread settings. You can use a few yeasts during the hot and humid months of summer.

Nutrition Info: Calories: 34 calories;Total Carbohydrate: 5.7 g ;Cholesterol: 1 mg ;Total Fat: 1 g ;Protein: 1 g ;Sodium: 313 mg

The Easiest Bread Maker Bread

Servings: 12
Cooking Time: 3 Hours
Ingredients:
- 1 cup lukewarm water
- 1/3 cup lukewarm milk
- 3 tablespoons butter, unsalted
- 3 3/4 cups unbleached all-purpose flour
- 3 tablespoons sugar
- 1 1/2 teaspoons salt
- 1 1/2 teaspoons active dry yeast

Directions:
1. Add liquid ingredients to the bread pan.
2. Measure and add dry ingredients (except yeast) to the bread pan.
3. Make a well in the center of the dry ingredients and add the yeast .
4. Snap the baking pan into the bread maker and close the lid.
5. Choose the Basic setting, preferred crust color and press Start.
6. When the loaf is done, remove the pan from the machine. After about 5 minutes, gently shake the pan to loosen the loaf and turn it out onto a rack to cool.
7. Store bread, well-wrapped, on the counter up to 4 days, or freeze for up to 3 months.

Nutrition Info: Calories: 183, Sodium: 316 mg, Dietary Fiber: 1.2 g, Fat: 3.3 g, Carbs: 33.3 g, Protein: 4.5 g.

Flax Bread

Servings: 8 Pcs
Cooking Time: 18 To 20 Minutes
Ingredients:
- ¾ cup of water
- 200 g ground flax seeds
- ½ cup psyllium husk powder
- 1 Tbsp. baking powder
- Seven large egg whites
- 3 Tbsp. butter
- 2 tsp. salt
- ¼ cup granulated stevia
- One large whole egg
- 1 ½ cups whey protein isolate

Directions:

1. Preheat the oven to 350F.
2. Combine whey protein isolate, psyllium husk, baking powder, sweetener, and salt.
3. In another bowl, mix the water, butter, egg
4. and egg whites.
5. Slowly add psyllium husk mixture to egg mixture and mix well.
6. Grease the pan lightly with butter and pour in the batter.
7. Bake in the oven until the bread is set, about 18 to 20 minutes.

Nutrition Info: Calories: 265.5;Fat: 15.68g;Carb: 1.88g;Protein:24.34 g

Homemade Hot Dog And Hamburger Buns

Servings: 8 - 10
Cooking Time: 1 Hour 35 Minutes
Ingredients:
- 1 1/4 cups milk, slightly warmed
- 1 egg, beaten
- 2 tablespoons butter, unsalted
- 1/4 cup white sugar
- 3/4 teaspoon salt
- 3 3/4 cups bread flour
- 1 1/4 teaspoons active dry yeast
- Flour, for surface

Directions:
1. Place all ingredients into the pan of the bread maker in the following order, reserving yeast: milk, egg, butter, sugar, salt, flour.
2. Make a well in the center of the dry ingredients and add the yeast.
3. Select Dough cycle. When cycle is complete, turn out onto floured surface.
4. Cut dough in half and roll each half out to a 1" thick circle.
5. Cut each half into 6 (3 1/2") rounds with inverted glass as a cutter. (For hot dog buns, cut lengthwise into 1-inch-thick rolls, and cut a slit along the length of the bun for easier separation later.)
6. Place on a greased baking sheet far apart and brush with melted butter.
7. Cover and let rise until doubled, about one hour; preheat an oven to 350°F.
8. Bake for 9 minutes.

9. Let cool and serve with your favorite meats and toppings!

Nutrition Info: Calories: 233, Sodium: 212 mg, Dietary Fiber: 1.4 g, Fat: 3.8 g, Carbs: 42.5 g, Protein: 6.6 g.

Soft Egg Bread

Servings: 1 Loaf
Cooking Time: 10 Minutes
Ingredients:

- 16 slice bread (2 pounds)
- 1 cup milk, at 80°F to 90°F
- 5 tablespoons melted butter, cooled
- 3 eggs, at room temperature
- ⅓ cup sugar
- 2 teaspoons salt
- 4 cups white bread flour
- 1 cup oat bran
- 3 cups whole-wheat bread flour
- 1½ teaspoons bread machine or instant yeast

Directions:
1. Preparing the Ingredients.
2. Place the ingredients in your bread machine as recommended by the manufacturer.
3. Select the Bake cycle
4. Turn on the bread maker. Select the White / Basic setting, then select the dough size and medium crust. Press Start.
5. When this is done, and the bread is baked, remove the pan from the machine. Let stand a few minutes.
6. Remove the bread from the pan and leave it on a wire rack to cool for at least 10 minutes. Slice and serve.

Italian Ciabatta

Servings: 2 Loaves
Cooking Time: 25 Minutes
Ingredients:

- 1½ cups water
- 1½ teaspoons salt
- 1teaspoon white sugar
- 1tablespoon olive oil
- 3¼ cups bread flour
- 1½ teaspoons bread machine yeast

Directions:
1. Place the ingredients into the pan of the bread machine in the order suggested by the manufacturer. Select the Dough cycle, and Start. Carefully measure the ingredients into the pan.
2. When the cycle is completed, the dough will be a sticky and wet. Do not add more flour. Place the dough on a generously floured board, cover with a large bowl, and let it rest for 15 minutes.
3. Select your bread machine's program to ITALIAN BREAD / SANDWICH mode and choose the crust color to MEDIUM.
4. Lightly flour baking sheets or line them with parchment paper. Using a knife, divide the dough into 2 pieces, and form each into a 3x14-inch oval. Place the loaves on a sheet and dust it lightly with some flour. Cover it, and let it rise in a draft-free place for approximately 45 minutes.
5. Spritz the loaves with water. Place the loaves in the oven, positioned on the middle rack. Bake until golden brown, 25 to 30 minutes.
6. Serve and enjoy!

Nutrition Info: Calories 73;Total Fat 0.9g;Cholesterol 0 mg;Sodium 146.3 mg;Total Carbohydrate 13.7g

Banana Lemon Loaf

Servings: 1 Loaf (16 Slices)
Cooking Time: 1 Hour And 30 Minutes
Ingredients:

- 2 cups all-purpose flour
- 1 cup bananas, very ripe and mashed
- 1 cup walnuts, chopped
- 1 cup of sugar
- One tablespoon baking powder
- One teaspoon lemon peel, grated
- ½ teaspoon salt
- Two eggs
- ½ cup of vegetable oil
- Two tablespoons lemon juice

Directions:
1. Put all ingredients into a pan in this order: bananas, wet ingredients, and then dry ingredients.
2. Press the "Quick" or "Cake" setting of your bread machine.
3. Allow the cycles to be completed.

4. Take out the pan from the machine. The cooldown for 10 minutes before slicing the bread enjoy.

Nutrition Info: Calories: 120;Carbohydrates: 15g;Fat: 6g;Protein: 2g

Honey White Bread

Servings: 1 Loaf
Cooking Time: 15 Minutes
Ingredients:
- 1 cup milk
- Three tablespoons unsalted butter, melted
- Two tablespoons honey
- 3 cups bread flour
- 3/4 teaspoon salt
- 3/4 teaspoon vitamin c powder
- 3/4 teaspoon ground ginger
- 1 1/2 teaspoons active dry yeast

Directions:
1. Follow the order as directed in your bread machine manual on how to assemble the ingredients. Use the setting for the Basic Bread cycle.

Nutrition Info: Calories: 172 Cal;Carbohydrates: 28.9 g;Cholesterol: 9 mg;Fat: 3.9 g;Protein: 5 g

Multigrain Olive Oil White Bread

Servings: 1 Loaf (16 Slices)
Cooking Time: 1 Hour And 30 Minutes
Ingredients:
- For the Dough
- 300 ml water
- 500 grams bakers flour
- 8 grams dried yeast
- 10 ml salt
- 5 ml caster suger
- 40 ml olive oil
- For the Seed mix
- 40 grams sunflower seeds
- 20 grams sesame seeds
- 20 grams flax seeds
- 20 grams quinoa
- 20 grams pumpkin seeds

Directions:
1. For the water: to 100ml of boiling water add 200ml of cold water.

2. Add the ingredients in the order required by the manufacturer.
3. add the seeds at the time required by your machine.
4. Empty dough onto a floured surface and gently use your finger tips to push some of the air out of it. Shape however you like and place on or in an oiled baking tray. Sprinkle with flour or brush with egg for a glazed finish. Slash the top. Cover and rise for 30 mins.
5. Heat oven to 240C/220C fan/gas 8. Bake for 30-35 mins until browned and crisp.

Nutrition Info: Calories 114.1;Total Fat 3.1 g;Saturated Fat 0.5 g;Polyunsaturated Fat 0.4 g;Monounsaturated Fat 1.9 g;Sodium 83.4 mg;Potassium 0.0 mg;Total Carbohydrate 19.7 g

Pretzel Rolls

Servings: 4
Cooking Time: 3 Hours 10 Minutes
Ingredients:
- 1 cup warm water
- 1 egg white, beaten
- 2 tablespoons oil
- 3 cups all-purpose flour
- 1/2 teaspoon salt
- 1 tablespoon granulated sugar
- 1 package dry yeast
- Coarse sea salt, for topping
- 1/3 cup baking soda (for boiling process, *DO NOT PUT IN THE PRETZEL DOUGH*)
- Flour, for surface

Directions:
1. Place the ingredients in bread machine pan in the order listed above, reserving yeast
2. Make a well in the center of the dry ingredients and add the yeast.
3. Select Dough cycle and press Start.
4. Remove the dough out onto a lightly floured surface and divide dough into four parts.
5. Roll the four parts into balls.
6. Place on greased cookie sheet and let rise uncovered for about 20 minutes or until puffy.
7. In a 3-quart saucepan, combine 2 quarts of water and baking soda and bring to a boil.
8. Preheat an oven to 425°F.

9. Lower 2 pretzels into the saucepan and simmer for 10 seconds on each side.
10. Lift from water with a slotted spoon and return to greased cookie sheet; repeat with remaining pretzels.
11. Let dry briefly.
12. Brush with egg white and sprinkle with coarse salt.
13. Bake in preheated oven for 20 minutes or until golden brown.
14. Let cool slightly before serving.
Nutrition Info: Calories: 422, Sodium: 547 mg, Dietary Fiber: 2.9 g, Fat: 7.8 g, Carbs: 75.3 g, Protein: 11.3 g.

Mom's White Bread

Servings: 16 Slices
Cooking Time: 3 H.
Ingredients:
- 1 cup and 3 Tbsp water
- 2 Tbsp vegetable oil
- 1½ tsp salt
- 2 Tbsp sugar
- 3¼ cups white bread flour
- 2 tsp active dry yeast

Directions:
1. Add each ingredient to the bread machine in the order and at the temperature recommended by your bread machine manufacturer.
2. Close the lid, select the basic or white bread, medium crust setting on your bread machine, and press start.
3. When the bread machine has finished baking, remove the bread and put it on a cooling rack.

Extra Buttery White Bread

Servings: 16 Slices
Cooking Time: 3 H. 10 Min.
Ingredients:
- 1⅛ cups milk
- 4 Tbsp unsalted butter
- 3 cups bread flour
- 1½ Tbsp white granulated sugar
- 1½ tsp salt
- 1½ tsp bread machine yeast

Directions:
1. Soften the butter in your microwave.
2. Add each ingredient to the bread machine in the order and at the temperature recommended by your bread machine manufacturer.
3. Close the lid, select the basic or white bread, medium crust setting on your bread machine, and press start.
4. When the bread machine has finished baking, remove the bread and put it on a cooling rack.

Crusty French Bread

Servings: 1 Loaf
Cooking Time: 10 Minutes
Ingredients:
- 12 slice bread (1½ pound)
- 1 cup water, at 80°F to 90°F
- 1¼ tablespoons olive oil
- 2 tablespoons sugar
- 1¼ teaspoons salt
- 3 cups white bread flour
- 1¼ teaspoons bread machine or instant yeast, or flax seeds (optional)

Directions:
1. Preparing the Ingredients.
2. Place the ingredients in your bread machine as recommended by the manufacturer.
3. Select the Bake cycle
4. Program the machine for French bread, select light or medium crust, and press Start.
5. When this is done, and the bread is baked, remove the pan from the machine. Let stand a few minutes.
6. Remove the bread from the pan and leave it on a wire rack to cool for at least 10 minutes.

Low-carb Multigrain Bread

Servings: 1 Loaf
Cooking Time: 1 Hour And 30 Minutes
Ingredients:
- ¾ cup whole-wheat flour
- ¼ cup cornmeal
- ¼ cup oatmeal
- Two tablespoons 7-grain cereals
- Two tablespoons baking powder

- One teaspoon salt
- ¼ teaspoon baking soda
- ¾ cup of water
- ¼ cup of vegetable oil
- ¼ cup of orange juice
- Three tablespoons aquafaba

Directions:
1. In the bread pan, add the wet ingredients first, then the dry ingredients.
2. Press the "Quick" or "Cake" mode of your bread machine.
3. Wait until all cycles are through.
4. Remove the bread pan from the machine.
5. Let the bread rest for 10 minutes in the pan before taking it out to cool down further.
6. Slice the bread after an hour has passed.

Nutrition Info: Calories: 60;Carbohydrates: 9g;Fat: 2g;Protein: 1g

Italian Restaurant Style Breadsticks

Servings: 12 - 16
Cooking Time: 3 Hours
Ingredients:
- 1 1/2 cups warm water
- 2 tablespoons butter, unsalted and melted
- 4 1/4 cups bread flour
- 2 tablespoons sugar
- 1 tablespoon salt
- 1 package active dry yeast
- For the topping:
- 1 stick unsalted butter, melted
- 2 teaspoons garlic powder
- 1 teaspoons salt
- 1 teaspoon parsley

Directions:
1. Add wet ingredients to your bread maker pan.
2. Mix dry ingredients, except yeast, and add to pan.
3. Make a well in the center of the dry ingredients and add the yeast.
4. Set to Dough cycle and press Start.
5. When the dough is done, roll out and cut into strips; keep in mind that they will double in size after they have risen, so roll them out thinner than a typical breadstick to yield room for them to grow.
6. Place on a greased baking sheet.

7. Cover the dough with a light towel and let sit in a warm area for 45 minutes to an hour.
8. Preheat an oven to 400°F.
9. Bake breadsticks for 6 to 7 minutes.
10. Mix the melted butter, garlic powder, salt and parsley in a small mixing bowl.
11. Brush the bread sticks with half the butter mixture; return to oven and bake for 5 to 8 additional minutes.
12. Remove breadsticks from the oven and brush the other half of the butter mixture.
13. Allow to cool for a few minutes before serving.

Nutrition Info: Calories: 148, Sodium: 450 mg, Dietary Fiber: 1 g, Fat: 2.5 g, Carbs: 27.3 g, Protein: 3.7 g.

Peasant Bread

Servings: 12
Cooking Time: 3 Hours
Ingredients:
- 2 tablespoons full rounded yeast
- 2 cups white bread flour
- 1 1/2 tablespoons sugar
- 1 tablespoon salt
- 7/8 cup water
- For the topping:
- Olive oil
- Poppy seeds

Directions:
1. Add water first, then add the dry ingredients to the bread machine, reserving yeast.
2. Make a well in the center of the dry ingredients and add the yeast.
3. Choose French cycle, light crust color, and push Start.
4. When bread is finished, coat the top of loaf with a little olive oil and lightly sprinkle with poppy seeds.
5. Allow to cool slightly and serve warm with extra olive oil for dipping.

Nutrition Info: Calories: 87, Sodium: 583 mg, Dietary Fiber: 1 g, Fat: 0.3 g, Carbs: 18.2 g, Protein: 2.9 g.

Apricot Oat

Servings: 1 Loaf

Cooking Time: 25 Minutes
Ingredients:
- 4 1/4 cups bread flour
- 2/3 cup rolled oats
- One tablespoon white sugar
- Two teaspoons active dry yeast
- 1 1/2 teaspoons salt
- One teaspoon ground cinnamon
- Two tablespoons butter cut up
- 1 2/3 cups orange juice
- 1/2 cup diced dried apricots
- Two tablespoons honey, warmed

Directions:
1. Into the bread machine's pan, put the bread ingredients in the order suggested by the manufacturer. Then pout in dried apricots before the knead cycle completes.
2. Immediately remove bread from a machine when it's done and then glaze with warmed honey. Let to cool thoroughly before serving.

Nutrition Info: Calories: 80 calories;Total Carbohydrate: 14.4 g ;Cholesterol: 5 mg ;Total Fat: 2.3 g ;Protein: 1.3 g ;Sodium: 306 mg

Gluten-free White Bread

Servings: 14 Slices
Cooking Time: 3 H.
Ingredients:
- 2 eggs
- 1⅓ cups milk
- 6 Tbsp oil
- 1 tsp vinegar
- 3⅝ cups white bread flour
- 1 tsp salt
- 2 Tbsp sugar
- 2 tsp dove farm quick yeast

Directions:
1. Add each ingredient to the bread machine in the order and at the temperature recommended by your bread machine manufacturer.
2. Close the lid and start the machine on the gluten free bread program, if available. Alternatively use the basic or rapid setting with a dark crust option.
3. When the bread machine has finished baking, remove the bread and put it on a cooling rack.

Orange Date Bread

Servings: 1 Loaf
Cooking Time: 1 Hour And 30 Minutes
Ingredients:
- 2 cups all-purpose flour
- 1 cup dates, chopped
- ¾ cup of sugar
- ½ cup walnuts, chopped
- Two tablespoons orange rind, grated
- 1 ½ teaspoons baking powder
- One teaspoon baking soda
- ½ cup of orange juice
- ½ cup of water
- One tablespoon vegetable oil
- One teaspoon vanilla extract

Directions:
1. Put the wet ingredients then the dry ingredients into the bread pan.
2. Press the "Quick" or "Cake" mode of the bread machine.
3. Allow all cycles to be finished.
4. Remove the pan from the machine, but keep the bread in the pan for 10 minutes more.
5. Take out the bread from the pan, and let it cool down completely before slicing.

Nutrition Info: Calories: 80;Carbohydrates: 14g;Fat: 2g;Protein: 1g

Soft White Bread

Servings: 14 Slices
Cooking Time: 3 H.
Ingredients:
- 2 cups water
- 4 tsp yeast
- 6 Tbsp sugar
- ½ cup vegetable oil
- 2 tsp salt
- 3 cups strong white flour

Directions:
1. Add each ingredient to the bread machine in the order and at the temperature recommended by your bread machine manufacturer.
2. Close the lid, select the basic bread, low crust setting on your bread machine, and press start.

3. When the bread machine has finished baking, remove the bread and put it on a cooling rack.

Almond Flour Bread

Servings: 10 Pcs
Cooking Time: 10 Minutes
Ingredients:
- Four egg whites
- Two egg yolks
- 2 cups almond flour
- 1/4 cup butter, melted
- 2 tbsp psyllium husk powder
- 1 1/2 tbsp baking powder
- 1/2 tsp xanthan gum
- Salt
- 1/2 cup + 2 tbsp warm water
- 2 1/4 tsp yeast

Directions:
1. Use a mixing bowl to combine all of the dry ingredients except for the yeast.
2. In the bread machine pan, add all the wet ingredients.
3. Add all of your dry ingredients from the small mixing bowl to the bread machine pan.
4. Set the machine to the basic setting.
5. When the bread is finished, remove it to the machine pan from the bread machine.
6. Let cool slightly before transferring to a cooling rack.
7. It can be stored for four days on the counter and three months in the freezer.

Nutrition Info: Calories: 110 ;Carbohydrates: 2.4g ;Protein: 4g

All-purpose White Bread

Servings: 1 Loaf
Cooking Time: 40 Minutes
Ingredients:
- ¾ cup water at 80 degrees F
- One tablespoon melted butter cooled
- One tablespoon sugar
- ¾ teaspoon salt
- Two tablespoons skim milk powder
- 2 cups white bread flour
- ¾ teaspoon instant yeast

Directions:
1. Add all of the ingredients to your bread machine, carefully following the instructions of the manufacturer.
2. Set the program of your bread machine to Basic/White Bread and set crust type to Medium.
3. Press START.
4. Wait until the cycle completes.
5. Once the loaf is ready, take the bucket out and let the loaf cool for 5 minutes.
6. Gently shake the bucket to remove the loaf.
7. Put to a cooling rack, slice, and serve.

Nutrition Info: Calories: 140 Cal;Fat: 2 g ;Carbohydrates:27 g ;Protein: 44 g ;Fibre: 2 g

SOURDOUGH BREAD

Gluten-free Sourdough Bread

Servings: 12
Cooking Time: 5 Minutes
Ingredients:

- 1 cup water
- 3 eggs
- 3/4 cup ricotta cheese
- 1/4 cup honey
- 1/4 cup vegetable oil
- 1 teaspoon cider vinegar
- 3/4 cup gluten-free sourdough starter
- 2 cups white rice flour
- 2/3 cup potato starch
- 1/3 cup tapioca flour
- 1/2 cup dry milk powder
- 3 1/2 teaspoons xanthan gum
- 1 1/2 teaspoons salt

Directions:

1. Preparing the Ingredients.
2. Combine wet ingredients and pour into bread maker pan.
3. Mix together dry ingredients in a large mixing bowl, and add on top of the wet ingredients.
4. Select the Bake cycle
5. Select Gluten-Free cycle and press Start.
6. Remove the pan from the machine and allow the bread to remain in the pan for approximately 10 minutes.
7. Transfer to a cooling rack before slicing.

Pecan Apple Spice Bread

Servings: 1 Loaf
Cooking Time: 10 Minutes
Ingredients:

- 12 slice bread (1½ pounds)
- ⅓ cup lukewarm water
- 2¼ tablespoons canola oil
- ¾ teaspoon apple cider vinegar
- 2¼ tablespoons light brown sugar, packed
- ¾ cup Granny Smith apples, grated
- 2 eggs, room temperature, slightly beaten
- ½ cup nonfat dry milk powder
- ½ cup brown rice flour

- ½ cup tapioca flour
- ½ cup millet flour
- ⅓ cup corn starch
- 1½ tablespoons apple pie spice
- ¾ tablespoon xanthan gum
- ¾ teaspoon table salt
- 1¼ teaspoons bread machine yeast
- ⅓ cup pecans, chopped

Directions:

1. Preparing the Ingredients.
2. Choose the size of loaf of your preference and then measure the ingredients.
3. Add all of the ingredients mentioned previously in the list, close the lid after placing the pan in the bread machine.
4. Select the Bake cycle
5. Turn on the bread machine. Select the White/Basic setting, select the loaf size, and the crust color. Press start.
6. When the cycle is finished, carefully remove the pan from the bread maker and let rest. When the machine signals to add ingredients, add the chopped pecans.
7. Remove the bread from the pan, put in a wire rack to cool for at least 10 minutes, and slice.

Lemon Sourdough Bread

Servings: 1 Loaf
Cooking Time: 10 Minutes
Ingredients:

- 12 slice bread (1½ pounds)
- ¾ cup Simple Sourdough Starter (here) or No-Yeast Sourdough Starter (here), fed, active, and at room temperature
- ¾ cup water, at 80°F to 90°F
- 1 egg, at room temperature
- 3 tablespoons butter, melted and cooled
- ⅓ cup honey
- 1½ teaspoons salt
- 2 teaspoons lemon zest
- 1½ teaspoons lime zest
- ⅓ cup wheat germ
- 3 cups white bread flour
- 1¾ teaspoons bread machine or instant yeast

Directions:
1. Preparing the Ingredients.
2. Choose the size of loaf of your preference and then measure the ingredients.
3. Add all of the ingredients mentioned previously in the list, close the lid after placing the pan in the bread machine Select the Bake cycle.
4. Turn on the bread machine. Select the Whole-Wheat/Whole-Grain bread setting, select the loaf size, select light or medium crust. Press start.
5. When the cycle is finished, carefully remove the pan from the bread maker and let it rest.
6. Remove the bread from the pan, put in a wire rack to cool for at least 10 minutes, and slice.

Mix Seed Bread

Servings: 1 Loaf
Cooking Time: 10 Minutes
Ingredients:
- 12 slice bread (1½ pounds)
- 2 cups lukewarm milk
- 6 tablespoons cooking oil
- 1 teaspoon vinegar
- 2 eggs, slightly beaten
- 1 tablespoon sugar
- 1 teaspoon table salt
- 2⅔ cups gluten-free flour(s) of your choice
- 2 tablespoons poppy seeds
- 2 tablespoons pumpkin seeds
- 2 tablespoons sunflower seeds
- 2 teaspoons bread machine yeast

Directions:
1. Preparing the Ingredients.
2. Choose the size of loaf of your preference and then measure the ingredients.
3. Add all of the ingredients mentioned previously in the list, close the lid after placing the pan in the bread machine
4. Select the Bake cycle
5. Turn on the bread machine. Select the White/Basic setting, select the loaf size, and the crust color. Press start.
6. When the cycle is finished, carefully remove the pan from the bread maker and let it rest.
7. Remove the bread from the pan, put in a wire rack to cool for at least 10 minutes, and slice.

Multigrain Sourdough Bread

Servings: 1 Loaf
Cooking Time: 10 Minutes
Ingredients:
- 12 slice bread (1½ pounds)
- ⅔ cup water, at 80°F to 90°F
- ¾ cup Simple Sourdough Starter, fed, active, and at room temperature
- 2 tablespoons melted butter, cooled
- 2½ tablespoons sugar
- ¾ teaspoon salt
- ¾ cup multigrain cereal
- 2⅔ cups white bread flour
- 1½ teaspoons bread machine or instant yeast

Directions:
1. Preparing the Ingredients.
2. Choose the size of loaf of your preference and then measure the ingredients.
3. Add all of the ingredients mentioned previously in the list, close the lid after placing the pan in the bread machine.
4. Select the Bake cycle
5. Turn on the bread machine. Select the Wheat/Whole-Grain bread setting, select the loaf size, and the crust color. Press start. When the cycle is finished, carefully remove the pan from the bread maker and let it rest.
6. Remove the bread from the pan, put in a wire rack to cool for at least 10 minutes, and slice.

No-yeast Whole-wheat Sourdough Starter

Servings: 2 Cups (32 Servings)
Cooking Time: 10 Minutes Plus Fermenting Time
Ingredients:
- 1 cup whole-wheat flour, divided
- ½ teaspoon honey
- 1 cup chlorine-free bottled water, at room temperature, divided

Directions:
1. Preparing the Ingredients.
2. Stir together ½ cup of flour, ½ cup of water, and the honey in a large glass bowl with a wooden spoon. Loosely cover the bowl with plastic wrap and place it in a warm area for 5 days, stirring at least twice a day.

After 5 days, stir in the remaining ½ cup of flour and ½ cup of water.

3.   Select the Bake cycle

4.   Cover the bowl loosely again with plastic wrap and place it in a warm area.

5.   When the starter has bubbles and foam on top, it is ready to use.

6.   Store the starter in the refrigerator in a covered glass jar, and stir it before using. If you use half, replenish the starter with ½ cup flour and ½ cup water

San Francisco Sourdough Bread

Servings: 1 Loaf

Cooking Time: 10 Minutes

Ingredients:

- 12 slice bread (1½ pounds)
- 1 cup plus 2 tablespoons Simple Sourdough Starter (here) or No-Yeast Sourdough Starter (here), fed, active, and at room temperature
- ½ cup plus 1 tablespoon water, at 80°F to 90°F
- 2¼ tablespoons olive oil
- 1½ teaspoons salt
- 2 tablespoons sugar
- 1½ tablespoons skim milk powder
- ⅓ cup whole-wheat flour
- 2⅔ cups white bread flour
- 1⅔ teaspoons bread machine or instant yeast

Directions:

1.   Preparing the Ingredients.

2.   Choose the size of loaf of your preference and then measure the ingredients.

3.   Add all of the ingredients mentioned previously in the list, close the lid after placing the pan in the bread machine

4.   Select the Bake cycle

5.   Turn on the bread machine. Select the White/Basic setting, select the loaf size, and the crust color. Press start.

6.   When the cycle is finished, carefully remove the pan from the bread maker and let it rest.

7.   Remove the bread from the pan, put in a wire rack to cool for at least 10 minutes, and slice.

Basic Honey Bread

Servings: 1 Loaf

Cooking Time: 10 Minutes

Ingredients:

- 12 slice bread (1½ pounds)
- 1½ cups warm milk
- ¼ cup unsalted butter, melted
- 2 eggs, beaten
- 1 teaspoon apple cider vinegar
- ½ cup honey
- 1 teaspoon table salt
- 3 cups gluten-free flour(s) of your choice
- 1½ teaspoons xanthan gum
- 1¾ teaspoons bread machine yeast

Directions:

1.   Preparing the Ingredients.

2.   Choose the size of loaf of your preference and then measure the ingredients.

3.   Add all of the ingredients mentioned previously in the list, close the lid after placing the pan in the bread machine.

4.   Select the Bake cycle

5.   Turn on the bread machine. Select the White/Basic or Gluten-Free (if your machine has this setting) setting, select the loaf size, and the crust color. Press start.

6.   When the cycle is finished, carefully remove the pan from the bread maker and let it rest.

7.   Remove the bread from the pan, put in a wire rack to cool for at least 10 minutes, and slice.

Instant Cocoa Bread

Servings: 1 Loaf

Cooking Time: 10 Minutes

Ingredients:

- 12 slice bread (1½ pounds)
- 1⅛ cups lukewarm water
- 2 large eggs, beaten
- 2¼ tablespoons molasses
- 1½ tablespoons canola oil
- ¾ teaspoon apple cider vinegar
- 2¼ tablespoons light brown sugar
- 1⅛ teaspoons table salt
- 1½ cups white rice flour
- ½ cup potato starch

- ¼ cup tapioca flour
- 1½ teaspoons xanthan gum
- 1½ teaspoons cocoa powder
- 1½ teaspoons instant coffee granules
- 2 teaspoons bread machine yeast

Directions:

1. Preparing the Ingredients.
2. Choose the size of loaf of your preference and then measure the ingredients.
3. Add all of the ingredients mentioned previously in the list, close the lid after placing the pan in the bread machine Select the Bake cycle
4. Turn on the bread machine. Select the White/Basic or Gluten-Free (if your machine has this setting) setting, select the loaf size, select light or medium crust. Press start.
5. When the cycle is finished, carefully remove the pan from the bread maker and let it rest.
6. Remove the bread from the pan, put in a wire rack to cool for at least 10 minutes, and slice.

Sourdough Beer Bread

Servings: 1 Loaf

Cooking Time: 10 Minutes

Ingredients:

- 12 slice bread (1½ pounds)
- 1 cup Simple Sourdough Starter (here) or No-Yeast Sourdough Starter (here), fed, active, and at room temperature
- ½ cup plus 1 tablespoon dark beer, at 80°F to 90°F
- 1½ tablespoons melted butter, cooled
- ¾ tablespoon sugar
- 1⅛ teaspoons salt
- 2⅔ cups white bread flour
- 1⅛ teaspoons bread machine or instant yeast

Directions:

1. Preparing the Ingredients.
2. Choose the size of loaf of your preference and then measure the ingredients.
3. Add all of the ingredients mentioned previously in the list, close the lid after placing the pan in the bread machine
4. Select the Bake cycle

5. Turn on the bread machine. Select the Wheat/Whole-Grain bread setting, select the loaf size, and the crust color. Press start.
6. When the cycle is finished, carefully remove the pan from the bread maker and let it rest.
7. Remove the bread from the pan, put in a wire rack to cool for at least 10 minutes, and slice.

Pecan Cranberry Bread

Servings: 1 Loaf

Cooking Time: 10 Minutes

Ingredients:

- 12 slice bread (1½ pounds)
- 1⅛ cups lukewarm water
- 3 tablespoons canola oil
- ¾ tablespoon orange zest
- ¾ teaspoon apple cider vinegar
- 2 eggs, slightly beaten
- 2¼ tablespoons sugar
- ¾ teaspoon table salt
- 1½ cups white rice flour
- ½ cup nonfat dry milk powder
- ⅓ cup tapioca flour
- ⅓ cup potato starch
- ¼ cup corn starch
- ¾ tablespoon xanthan gum
- 1½ teaspoons bread machine yeast
- ½ cup dried cranberries
- ½ cup pecan pieces

Directions:

1. Preparing the Ingredients.
2. Choose the size of loaf of your preference and then measure the ingredients.
3. Add all of the ingredients mentioned previously in the list, close the lid after placing the pan in the bread machine. Select the Bake cycle
4. Turn on the bread maker. Select the Gluten Free or Fruit/Nut (if your machine has this setting) setting, then the loaf size, and finally the crust color. Start the cycle. (If you don't have either of the above settings, use Basic/White.).
5. When the machine signals to add ingredients, add the pecans and cranberries. (Some machines have a fruit/nut hopper where you can add the pecans and cranberries when you start the machine.

The machine will automatically add them to the dough during the baking process.).
6.   When the cycle is finished, carefully remove the pan from the bread maker and let it rest.
7.   Remove the bread from the pan, put in a wire rack to cool for at least 10 minutes, and slice.

Basic Sourdough Bread

Servings: 1 Loaf
Cooking Time: 10 Minutes
Ingredients:
- 12 slice bread (1½ pounds)
- 2 cups Simple Sourdough Starter (here), fed, active, and at room temperature
- 2 tablespoons water, at 80°F to 90°F
- ¾ teaspoon apple cider vinegar
- 1⅓ teaspoons sugar
- 1 teaspoon salt
- 1⅔ cups white bread flour
- ½ cup nonfat dry milk powder
- 1 teaspoon bread machine or instant yeast

Directions:
1.   Preparing the Ingredients.
2.   Choose the size of loaf of your preference and then measure the ingredients.
3.   Add all of the ingredients mentioned previously in the list, close the lid after placing the pan in the bread machine.
4.   Select the Bake cycle
5.   Turn on the bread machine. Select the White/Basic setting, select the loaf size, and the crust color. Press start.
6.   When the cycle is finished, carefully remove the pan from the bread maker and let rest. When the machine signals to add ingredients, add the chopped pecans.
7.   Remove the bread from the pan, put in a wire rack to cool for at least 5 minutes, and slice.

Garlic Parsley Bread

Servings: 1 Loaf
Cooking Time: 10 Minutes
Ingredients:
- 12 slice bread (1½ pounds)
- 1¼ cups almond or coconut milk

- 3 tablespoons flax meal
- ½ cup + 1 tablespoon warm water
- 3 tablespoons butter
- 2¼ tablespoons maple syrup
- 2¼ teaspoons apple cider vinegar
- 3 tablespoons parsley, loosely chopped
- 8–9 cloves garlic, minced
- ¾ teaspoon table salt
- 6 tablespoons + 2 teaspoons brown rice flour
- ⅓ cup corn starch
- 3 tablespoons potato starch
- 2 teaspoons xanthan gum
- 1½ tablespoons garlic powder
- 1½ tablespoons onion powder
- 1½ teaspoons bread machine yeast

Directions:
1.   Preparing the Ingredients.
2.   Combine the water and flax meal in a bowl; set aside for 5–10 minutes to mix well.
3.   Choose the size of loaf of your preference and then measure the ingredients.
4.   Add all of the ingredients mentioned previously in the list, including the flax meal. Close the lid after placing the pan in the bread machine.
5.   Select the Bake cycle
6.   Turn on the bread machine. Select the White/Basic or Gluten-Free (if your machine has this setting) setting, select the loaf size, select light or medium crust. Press start.
7.   When the cycle is finished, carefully remove the pan from the bread maker and let it rest.
8.   Remove the bread from the pan, put in a wire rack to cool for at least 10 minutes, and slice.

Sourdough Milk Bread

Servings: 1 Loaf
Cooking Time: 10 Minutes
Ingredients:
- 12 slice bread (1½ pounds)
- 1½ cups Simple Sourdough Starter (here) or No-Yeast Sourdough Starter (here), fed, active, and at room temperature
- ⅓ cup milk, at 80°F to 90°F
- 3 tablespoons olive oil
- 1½ tablespoons honey

- 1 teaspoon salt
- 3 cups white bread flour
- 1 teaspoon bread machine or instant yeast

Directions:
1. Preparing the Ingredients.
2. Choose the size of loaf of your preference and then measure the ingredients.
3. Add all of the ingredients mentioned previously in the list, close the lid after placing the pan in the bread machine.
4. Select the Bake cycle
5. Turn on the bread machine. Select the White/Basic setting, select the loaf size, and the crust color. Press start.
6. When the cycle is finished, carefully remove the pan from the bread maker and let it rest.
7. Remove the bread from the pan, put in a wire rack to cool for at least 10 minutes, and slice.

Dark Chocolate Sourdough

Servings: 1 Loaf
Cooking Time: 10 Minutes
Ingredients:
- 12 slice bread (1½ pounds)
- 2 cups No-Yeast Sourdough Starter, fed, active, and at room temperature
- 2 tablespoons water, at 80°F to 90°F
- 2 tablespoons melted butter, cooled
- ¾ teaspoon pure vanilla extract
- 2 teaspoons sugar
- 1½ teaspoons salt
- ⅓ teaspoon ground cinnamon
- ¼ cup unsweetened cocoa powder
- 2½ cups white bread flour
- 1½ teaspoons bread machine or instant yeast
- ½ cup semisweet chocolate chips
- ⅓ cup chopped pistachios
- ⅓ cup raisins

Directions:
1. Preparing the Ingredients.
2. Choose the size of loaf of your preference and then measure the ingredients.
3. Add all of the ingredients mentioned previously in the list, close the lid after placing the pan in the bread machine
4. Select the Bake cycle

5. Turn on the bread machine. Select the Wheat/Whole-Grain bread setting, select the loaf size, and the crust color. Press start. When the cycle is finished, carefully remove the pan from the bread maker and let it rest.
6. Remove the bread from the pan, put in a wire rack to cool for at least 5 minutes, and slice

Crusty Sourdough Bread

Servings: 1 Loaf
Cooking Time: 10 Minutes
Ingredients:
- 12 slice bread (1½ pounds)
- 1 cup Simple Sourdough Starter (here), fed, active, and at room temperature
- ½ cup water, at 80°F to 90°F
- 2 tablespoons honey
- 1½ teaspoons salt
- 3 cups white bread flour
- 1 teaspoon bread machine or instant yeast

Directions:
1. Preparing the Ingredients.
2. Choose the size of loaf of your preference and then measure the ingredients.
3. Add all of the ingredients mentioned previously in the list, close the lid after placing the pan in the bread machine
4. Select the Bake cycle
5. Turn on the bread machine. Select the Wheat/Whole-Grain bread setting, select the loaf size, and the crust color. Press start. When the cycle is finished, carefully remove the pan from the bread maker and let it rest.
6. Remove the bread from the pan, put in a wire rack to cool for at least 10 minutes, and slice.

No-yeast Sourdough Starter

Servings: 4 Cups
Cooking Time: 10 Minutes Plus Fermenting Time
Ingredients:
- 2 cups all-purpose flour
- 2 cups chlorine-free bottled water, at room temperature

Directions:
1. Preparing the Ingredients.

2. Stir together the flour and water in a large glass bowl with a wooden spoon. Loosely cover the bowl with plastic wrap and place it in a warm area for 3 to 4 days, stirring at least twice a day, or until bubbly.

3. Select the Bake cycle

4. Store the starter in the refrigerator in a covered glass jar, and stir it before using.

5. Replenish your starter by adding back the same amount you removed, in equal parts flour and water.

Pumpkin Jalapeno Bread

Servings: 1 Loaf
Cooking Time: 10 Minutes
Ingredients:

- 12 slice bread (1½ pounds)
- ½ cup lukewarm water
- 2 medium eggs, beaten
- ⅓ cup pumpkin puree
- 2¼ tablespoons honey
- 1½ tablespoons vegetable oil
- ¾ teaspoon apple cider vinegar
- 1½ teaspoons sugar
- ¾ teaspoon table salt
- ½ cup brown rice flour
- ½ cup tapioca flour
- ⅓ cup corn starch
- ⅓ cup yellow cornmeal
- ¾ tablespoon xanthan gum
- 1 small jalapeno pepper, seeded and deveined
- 1½ teaspoons crushed red pepper flakes
- 1¼ teaspoons bread machine yeast

Directions:

1. Preparing the Ingredients.

2. Choose the size of loaf of your preference and then measure the ingredients.

3. Add all of the ingredients mentioned previously in the list, close the lid after placing the pan in the bread machine.

4. Select the Bake cycle

5. Turn on the bread machine. Select the White/Basic setting, select the loaf size, and the crust color. Press start.

6. When the cycle is finished, carefully remove the pan from the bread maker and let rest. When the machine signals to add ingredients, add the chopped pecans.

7. Remove the bread from the pan, put in a wire rack to cool for at least 10 minutes, and slice.

Potica

Servings: 10 Servings
Cooking Time: 20 Minutes
Ingredients:

- Bread dough
- ½ cup milk
- ¼ cup cold butter, cut into small pieces
- 1 egg
- 2 cups bread flour
- ¼ cup sugar
- ¼ teaspoon salt
- 1 teaspoon bread machine yeast or fast-acting dry yeast filling
- 2 cups finely chopped or ground walnuts (about 7 oz)
- 1/3 cup honey
- 1/3 cup milk
- 3 tablespoons sugar
- 1 egg white, beaten

Directions:

1. Preparing the Ingredients.

2. Measure carefully, placing all bread dough ingredients in bread machine pan in the order recommended by the manufacturer.

3. Select the Bake cycle

4. Select Dough/Manual cycle. Do not use delay cycle. Remove dough from pan, using lightly floured hands. Cover and let rest 10 minutes on lightly floured surface. In small saucepan, combine all filling ingredients except egg white. Bring to a boil over medium heat, stirring frequently. Reduce heat; simmer uncovered 5 minutes, stirring occasionally.

5. Spread in shallow dish; cover and refrigerate until chilled.

6. Grease large cookie sheet with shortening. Roll dough into 16×12-inch rectangle on lightly floured surface. Spread filling over dough to within ½ inch of edges. Starting with 16-inch side, roll up tightly; pinch seam to seal. Stretch and shape roll until even. Coil roll of dough to form a snail shape. Place on

cookie sheet. Cover and let rise in warm place 30 to 60 minutes or until doubled in size. Dough is ready if indentation remains when touched.

7.   Heat oven to 325°F. Brush egg white over dough. Bake 45 to 55 minutes or until golden brown. Remove from cookie sheet to cooling rack.

Sourdough Cheddar Bread

Servings: 1 Loaf
Cooking Time: 10 Minutes
Ingredients:
- 12 slice bread (1½ pounds)
- 1 cup Simple Sourdough Starter or No-Yeast Sourdough Starter, fed, active, and at room temperature
- ⅓ cup water, at 80°F to 90°F
- 4 teaspoons sugar
- 1 teaspoon salt
- ½ cup (2 ounces) grated aged Cheddar cheese
- ⅔ cup whole-wheat flour
- ¼ cup oat bran
- 1⅓ cups white bread flour
- 1½ teaspoons bread machine or instant yeast

Directions:
1.   Preparing the Ingredients.
2.   Choose the size of loaf of your preference and then measure the ingredients.
3.   Add all of the ingredients mentioned previously in the list, close the lid after placing the pan in the bread machine
4.   Select the Bake cycle
5.   Turn on the bread machine. Select the Wheat/Whole-Grain bread setting, select the loaf size, and the crust color. Press start. When the cycle is finished, carefully remove the pan from the bread maker and let it rest.
6.   Remove the bread from the pan, put in a wire rack to cool for at least 5 minutes, and slice.

SPECIALTY BREAD

Brown Rice Flour Bread

Servings: 16
Cooking Time: 3 Hours And 48 Minutes
Ingredients:
- Water – 1 ½ cups
- Oil – 3 tbsp.
- Honey – 3 tbsp.
- Sea salt – 1 tsp.
- Xanthan gum – 1 tbsp.
- Brown rice flour – 2 ¾ cups
- Tapioca flour – ¾ cup
- Active dry yeast – 2 ¼ tsp.

Directions:
1. Add everything according to bread machine recommendations.
2. Select Whole Wheat cycle and press Start.
3. Remove the bread when done.
4. Cool, slice, and serve.

Nutrition Info: (Per Serving): Calories: 286; Total Fat: 3.3 g; Saturated Fat: 0.5 g; Carbohydrates: 58.6 g; Cholesterol: 0 mg; Fiber: 2.5 g; Calcium: 22 mg; Sodium: 148 mg; Protein: 2.2 g

Dry Fruit Cinnamon Bread

Servings: 1 Loaf
Ingredients:
- 16 slice bread (2 pounds)
- 1⅔ cups lukewarm milk
- ⅓ cup unsalted butter, melted
- ⅔ teaspoon pure vanilla extract
- ¼ teaspoon pure almond extract
- ⅓ cup light brown sugar
- 1⅓ teaspoons table salt
- 2 teaspoons ground cinnamon
- 4 cups white bread flour
- 1⅔ teaspoons bread machine yeast
- ⅔ cup dried mixed fruit
- ⅔ cup golden raisins, chopped
- 12 slice bread (1½ pounds)
- 1¼ cups lukewarm milk
- ¼ cup unsalted butter, melted
- ½ teaspoon pure vanilla extract
- ¼ teaspoon pure almond extract
- 3 tablespoons light brown sugar
- 1 teaspoon table salt
- 2 teaspoons ground cinnamon
- 3 cups white bread flour
- 1 teaspoon bread machine yeast
- ½ cup dried mixed fruit
- ½ cup golden raisins, chopped

Directions:
1. Choose the size of loaf you would like to make and measure your ingredients.
2. Add all of the ingredients except for the mixed fruit and raisins to the bread pan in the order listed above.
3. Place the pan in the bread machine and close the lid.
4. Turn on the bread maker. Select the White/Basic or Fruit/Nut (if your machine has this setting) setting, then the loaf size, and finally the crust color. Start the cycle.
5. When the machine signals to add ingredients, add the mixed fruit and raisins. (Some machines have a fruit/nut hopper where you can add the mixed fruit and raisins when you start the machine. The machine will automatically add them to the dough during the baking process.)
6. When the cycle is finished and the bread is baked, carefully remove the pan from the machine. Use a potholder as the handle will be very hot. Let rest for a few minutes.
7. Remove the bread from the pan and allow to cool on a wire rack for at least 10 minutes before slicing.

Nutrition Info: (Per Serving):Calories 193, fat 4.7 g, carbs 29.3 g, sodium 226 mg, protein 5 g

Low-sodium White Bread

Servings: 12
Cooking Time: 3 Hours And 25 Minutes
Ingredients:
- Water – 1 ¼ cup
- Oil – 2 tbsp.
- Vital wheat gluten – 1 ½ tsp.
- Sugar – 2 tbsp.
- White bread flour 3 ¼ cups
- Active dry yeast – 2 tsp.

- No sodium baking powder – 3 tsp.
- Butter – 1 tbsp., unsalted

Directions:
1. Add everything according to bread machine recommendations.
2. Select Basic bread, and Medium crust.
3. Remove the bread when done.
4. Cool, slice, and serve.

Nutrition Info: (Per Serving): Calories: 159; Total Fat: 2.6 g; Saturated Fat: 0.5 g; Carbohydrates: 29.1 g; Cholesterol: 0 mg; Fiber: 1.2 g; Calcium: 60 mg; Sodium: 3 mg; Protein: 4.8 g

Low-carb Carrot Bread

Servings: 15
Cooking Time: 3 Hours And 25 Minutes
Ingredients:
- Coconut flour - ½ cup
- Xanthan gum - 1/8 tsp.
- Baking powder - ½ tsp.
- Baking soda - ½ tsp.
- Salt - 1/4 tsp.
- Cinnamon - 2 tsp.
- Ginger - ½ tsp.
- Nutmeg - ¼ tsp.
- Granulated sweetener - 2 tbsp.
- Unsweetened almond milk - 1/3 cup
- Butter - ½ cup, melted
- Vanilla extract - 1 tsp.
- Maple extract - 1 tsp.
- Apple cider vinegar - ½ tsp.
- Eggs – 4
- Shredded carrots – 1 ounce

Directions:
1. Add everything in the order recommended by the machine manufacturer.
2. Select Basic bread and crust color. Press Start.
3. Remove the bread when done.
4. Slice, cool, and serve.

Nutrition Info: (Per Serving): Calories: 132; Total Fat: 9.4 g; Saturated Fat: 5.9 g; Carbohydrates: 8.8 g; Cholesterol: 60 mg; Fiber: 5.9 g; Calcium: 27 mg; Sodium: 198 mg; Protein: 4.1 g

Holiday Chocolate Bread

Servings: 1 Loaf
Ingredients:

- 16 slice bread (2 pounds)
- 1 cup + 3 tablespoons lukewarm milk
- 1 egg, at room temperature
- 2 tablespoons unsalted butter, melted
- 1½ teaspoons pure vanilla extract
- 2⅔ tablespoons sugar
- 1 teaspoon table salt
- 4 cups white bread flour
- 1⅓ teaspoons bread machine yeast
- ⅔ cup white chocolate chips
- ½ cup dried cranberries
- 12 slice bread (1½ pounds)
- ⅞ cup lukewarm milk
- 1 egg, at room temperature
- 1½ tablespoons unsalted butter, melted
- 1 teaspoon pure vanilla extract
- 2 tablespoons sugar
- ¾ teaspoon table salt
- 3 cups white bread flour
- 1 teaspoon bread machine yeast
- ½ cup white chocolate chips
- ⅓ cup dried cranberries

Directions:
1. Choose the size of loaf you would like to make and measure your ingredients.
2. Add all of the ingredients except for the chocolate chips and cranberries to the bread pan in the order listed above.
3. Place the pan in the bread machine and close the lid.
4. Turn on the bread maker. Select the White/Basic or Fruit/Nut (if your machine has this setting) setting, then the loaf size, and finally the crust color. Start the cycle.
5. When the machine signals to add ingredients, add the chocolate chips and cranberries. (Some machines have a fruit/nut hopper where you can add the chocolate chips and cranberries when you start the machine. The machine will automatically add them to the dough during the baking process.)
6. When the cycle is finished and the bread is baked, carefully remove the pan from the machine. Use a potholder as the handle will be very hot. Let rest for a few minutes.
7. Remove the bread from the pan and allow to cool on a wire rack for at least 10 minutes before slicing.

Nutrition Info: (Per Serving):Calories 204, fat 4.6 g, carbs 31.7 g, sodium 164 mg, protein 4.5 g

Challah Bread

Servings: 1 Loaf

Ingredients:
- 16 slice bread (2 pounds)
- 1 cup +¾ teaspoon water, lukewarm between 80 and 90⁰F
- 2 ½ tablespoons unsalted butter, melted
- 2 small eggs, beaten
- 2 ½ tablespoons sugar
- 1 ¾ teaspoons salt
- 4 ½ cups white bread flour
- 2 teaspoons bread machine yeast or rapid rise yeast
- 12 slice bread (1 ½ pounds)
- ¾ cup +1 tablespoon water, lukewarm between 80 and 90⁰F
- 2 tablespoons unsalted butter, melted
- 1 egg, beaten
- 2 tablespoons sugar
- 1 ½ teaspoons salt
- 3 ¼ cups white bread flour
- 1 ½ teaspoons bread machine yeast or rapid rise yeast
- For oven baking
- 1 egg yolk
- 2 tablespoons cold water
- 1 tablespoon poppy seed (optional)

Directions:
1. Choose the size of loaf you would like to make and measure your ingredients.
2. Add the ingredients to the bread pan in the order listed above.
3. Place the pan in the bread machine and close the lid.
4. Turn on the bread maker. Select the Dough setting, then the loaf size, and finally the crust color. Start the cycle.
5. Lightly flour a working surface and prepare a large baking sheet by greasing it with cooking spray or vegetable oil or line with parchment paper or a silicone mat.
6. Preheat the oven to 375°F and place the oven rack in the middle position.

7. After the dough cycle is done, carefully remove the dough from the pan and place it on the working surface. Divide dough in three even parts.
8. Roll each part into 13-inch-long cables for the 1 ½ pound Challah bread or 17-inch for the 2-pound loaf. Arrange the dough cables side by side and start braiding from its middle part.
9. In order to make a seal, pinch ends and tuck the ends under the braid.
10. Arrange the loaf onto the baking sheet; cover the sheet with a clean kitchen towel. Let rise for 45-60 minutes or more until it doubles in size.
11. In a mixing bowl, mix the egg yolk and cold water to make an egg wash. Gently brush the egg wash over the loaf. Sprinkle top with the poppy seed, if desired.
12. Bake for about 25-30 minutes or until loaf turns golden brown and is fully cooked.

Nutrition Info: (Per Serving):Calories 196, fat 3.3g, carbs 33.5 g, sodium 207, protein 6.4g

Cherry Christmas Bread

Servings: 1 Loaf

Ingredients:
- 16 slice bread (2 pounds)
- 1 cup + 1 tablespoon lukewarm milk
- 1 egg, at room temperature
- 2 tablespoons unsalted butter, melted
- 3 tablespoons light brown sugar
- ⅛ teaspoon ground cinnamon
- 4 cups white bread flour, divided
- 1½ teaspoons bread machine yeast
- ⅔ cup candied cherries
- ½ cup chopped almonds
- ½ cup raisins, chopped
- 12 slice bread (1½ pounds)
- ¾ cup lukewarm milk
- 1 egg, at room temperature
- 1½ tablespoons unsalted butter, melted
- 2¼ tablespoons light brown sugar
- ⅛ teaspoon ground cinnamon
- 3 cups white bread flour, divided
- 1⅛ teaspoons bread machine yeast
- ½ cup candied cherries
- ⅓ cup chopped almonds
- ⅓ cup raisins, chopped

Directions:

1. Choose the size of loaf you would like to make and measure your ingredients.
2. Add all of the ingredients except for the cherries, raisins, and almonds to the bread pan in the order listed above.
3. Place the pan in the bread machine and close the lid.
4. Turn on the bread maker. Select the White/Basic or Fruit/Nut (if your machine has this setting) setting, then the loaf size, and finally the crust color. Start the cycle.
5. When the machine signals to add ingredients, add the cherries, raisins, and almonds. (Some machines have a fruit/nut hopper where you can add the cherries, raisins, and almonds when you start the machine. The machine will automatically add them to the dough during the baking process.)
6. When the cycle is finished and the bread is baked, carefully remove the pan from the machine. Use a potholder as the handle will be very hot. Let rest for a few minutes.
7. Remove the bread from the pan and allow to cool on a wire rack for at least 10 minutes before slicing.

Nutrition Info: (Per Serving):Calories 176, fat 4.2 g, carbs 32.7 g, sodium 46 mg, protein 5.1 g

Coffee Caraway Seed Bread

Servings: 1 Loaf

Ingredients:
- 16 slice bread (2 pounds)
- 1 cup lukewarm water
- ½ cup brewed coffee, lukewarm
- 2 tablespoons balsamic vinegar
- 2 tablespoons olive oil
- 2 tablespoons dark molasses
- 1 tablespoon light brown sugar
- 1 teaspoon table salt
- 2 teaspoons caraway seeds
- ¼ cup unsweetened cocoa powder
- 1 cup dark rye flour
- 2½ cups white bread flour
- 2 teaspoons bread machine yeast
- 12 slice bread (1½ pounds)
- ¾ cup lukewarm water
- ⅓ cup brewed coffee, lukewarm
- 1½ tablespoons balsamic vinegar
- 1½ tablespoons olive oil

- 1½ tablespoons dark molasses
- ¾ tablespoon light brown sugar
- ¾ teaspoon table salt
- 1½ teaspoons caraway seeds
- 3 tablespoons unsweetened cocoa powder
- ¾ cup dark rye flour
- 1¾ cups white bread flour
- 1½ teaspoons bread machine yeast

Directions:
1. Choose the size of loaf you would like to make and measure your ingredients.
2. Add the ingredients to the bread pan in the order listed above.
3. Place the pan in the bread machine and close the lid.
4. Turn on the bread maker. Select the Whole Wheat/Wholegrain setting, then the loaf size, and finally the crust color. Start the cycle.
5. When the cycle is finished and the bread is baked, carefully remove the pan from the machine. Use a potholder as the handle will be very hot. Let rest for a few minutes.
6. Remove the bread from the pan and allow to cool down on a wire rack for at least 10 minutes or more before slicing.

Nutrition Info: (Per Serving):Calories 126, fat 1.8 g, carbs 22.6 g, sodium 148 mg, protein 4 g

Milk Honey Sourdough Bread

Servings: 1 Loaf

Ingredients:
- 16 slice bread (2 pounds)
- ½ cup lukewarm milk
- 2 cups sourdough starter
- ¼ cup olive oil
- 2 tablespoons honey
- 1⅓ teaspoons salt
- 4 cups white bread flour
- 1⅓ teaspoons bread machine yeast
- 12 slice bread (1½ pounds)
- ⅓ cup lukewarm milk
- 1½ cups sourdough starter
- 3 tablespoons olive oil
- 1½ tablespoons honey
- 1 teaspoon salt
- 3 cups white bread flour
- 1 teaspoon bread machine yeast

Directions:

1.   Choose the size of loaf you would like to make and measure your ingredients.
2.   Add the ingredients to the bread pan in the order listed above.
3.   Place the pan in the bread machine and close the lid.
4.   Turn on the bread maker. Select the White/Basic setting, then the loaf size, and finally the crust color. Start the cycle.
5.   When the cycle is finished and the bread is baked, carefully remove the pan from the machine. Use a potholder as the handle will be very hot. Let rest for a few minutes.
6.   Remove the bread from the pan and allow to cool on a wire rack for at least 10 minutes before slicing.

Nutrition Info: (Per Serving):Calories 186, fat 3.7 g, carbs 32.2 g, sodium 207 mg, protein 4 g

Cinnamon Beer Bread

Servings: 1 Loaf

Ingredients:

- 16 slice bread (2 pounds)
- 2 cups beer, at room temperature
- 1 cup unsalted butter, melted
- ⅓ cup honey
- 4 cups all-purpose flour
- 1⅓ teaspoons table salt
- ⅓ teaspoon ground cinnamon
- 1⅓ tablespoons baking powder
- 12 slice bread (1½ pounds)
- 1½ cups beer, at room temperature
- ⅓ cup unsalted butter, melted
- ¼ cup honey
- 3 cups all-purpose flour
- 1 teaspoon table salt
- ¼ teaspoon ground cinnamon
- 1 tablespoon baking powder

Directions:

1.   Choose the size of loaf you would like to make and measure your ingredients.
2.   Add the ingredients to the bread pan in the order listed above.
3.   Place the pan in the bread machine and close the lid.

4.   Turn on the bread maker. Select the Quick/Rapid setting, then the loaf size, and finally the crust color. Start the cycle.
5.   When the cycle is finished and the bread is baked, carefully remove the pan from the machine. Use a potholder as the handle will be very hot. Let rest for a few minutes.
6.   Remove the bread from the pan and allow to cool on a wire rack for at least 10 minutes before slicing.

Nutrition Info: (Per Serving):Calories 186, fat 4.6 g, carbs 26.4 g, sodium 217 mg, protein 3.5 g

No-salt White Bread

Servings: 12

Cooking Time: 3 Hours And 25 Minutes

Ingredients:

- Warm water - 1 cup
- Olive oil – 1 tbsp.
- Sugar – 1 ¼ tsp.
- Yeast – 1 ¼ tsp.
- Flour – 3 ¼ cup
- Egg white - 1

Directions:

1.   Dissolve the sugar in the water.
2.   Add yeast to the sugar water.
3.   Put flour, yeast mixture, and oil into the bread-maker.
4.   Select Basic bread setting.
5.   Add the egg white after 5 minutes.
6.   Remove the bread when it is done.
7.   Cool, slice, and serve.

Nutrition Info: (Per Serving): Calories: 275.3; Total Fat: 3 g; Saturated Fat: 0.4 g; Carbohydrates: 52.9 g; Cholesterol: 0 mg; Fiber: 2 g; Calcium: 22 mg; Sodium: 12.2 mg; Protein: 7.9 g

Low-sodium Bread

Servings: 12

Cooking Time: 3 Hours And 25 Minutes

Ingredients:

- Warm water – 1 cup
- Unsalted butter – 2 tbsp.
- Dry milk – 1 tbsp.
- All-purpose flour – 3 cups
- Bread machine yeast – 1 tsp.

Directions:

1. Add everything according to bread machine recommendations.
2. Select Basic cycle and crust color.
3. Remove the bread when done.
4. Cool, slice, and serve.

Nutrition Info: (Per Serving): Calories: 143.9; Total Fat: 2.7 g; Saturated Fat: 1.4 g; Carbohydrates: 25.1 g; Cholesterol: 5.8 mg; Fiber: 0.8 g; Calcium: 28 mg; Sodium: 3.5 mg; Protein: 4.3 g

Whole Grain Salt-free Bread

Servings: 16
Cooking Time: 3 Hours And 25 Minutes
Ingredients:
- Whole-grain cereal – 2/3 cup
- Water – 1 cup, boiling hot
- Oil – 2 tsp.
- Honey – 4 tsp.
- Orange zest of 1 orange
- Whole wheat flour – 2 cups
- Vital wheat gluten – 4 tsp.
- Active dry yeast – 2 ¼ tsp.

Directions:
1. Add everything in the bread pan in the order listed.
2. Select White/Basic setting. Use the Delay future.
3. Remove the bread when done.
4. Cool, sliced, and serve.

Nutrition Info: (Per Serving): Calories: 79; Total Fat: 0.8 g; Saturated Fat: 0.1 g; Carbohydrates: 15.3 g; Cholesterol: 0 mg; Fiber: 0.8 g; Calcium: 5 mg; Sodium: 1 mg; Protein: 2.7 g

Potato And Rice Flour Bread

Servings: 20
Cooking Time: 2 Hours And 10 Minutes
Ingredients:
- Eggs - 3
- Cider vinegar - 1 tsp.
- Oil - ¼ cup
- Water – 1 ½ cups
- White rice flour - 2 cups
- Potato starch - ½ cup

- Tapioca flour - ½ cup
- Cornstarch - 1/3 cup
- Xanthan gum - 1 tbsp.
- Sugar - 3 tbsp.
- Salt - 1 tsp.
- Milk powder - 2/3 cup (non-fat dry)
- Active dry yeast – 2 ¼ tsp.

Directions:
1. Add everything according to bread machine recommendations.
2. Select a Gluten-Free or Normal cycle.
3. Remove the bread when done.
4. Cool, slice, and serve.

Nutrition Info: (Per Serving): Calories: 144; Total Fat: 3.6 g; Saturated Fat: 0.5 g; Carbohydrates: 24.3 g; Cholesterol: 25 mg; Fiber: 0.7 g; Calcium: 59 mg; Sodium: 158 mg; Protein: 3.6 g

Milk And Honey Bread

Servings: 12
Cooking Time: 2 Hours And 10 Minutes
Ingredients:
- Warm milk – 1 ½ cups
- Unsalted butter – ¼ cup
- Eggs – 2, beaten
- Apple cider vinegar – 1 tsp.
- Honey – ½ cup
- All-purpose gluten-free flour – 3 cups
- Salt – 1 tsp.
- Xanthan gum – 1 ½ tsp
- Instant yeast – 1 ¾ tsp.

Directions:
1. Add everything according to bread machine recommendations.
2. Select Gluten-Free setting.
3. Remove the bread when done.
4. Cool, slice, and serve.

Nutrition Info: (Per Serving): Calories: 212; Total Fat: 6 g; Saturated Fat: 3 g; Carbohydrates: 35 g; Cholesterol: 40 mg; Fiber: 3 g; Calcium: 61 mg; Sodium: 263 mg; Protein: 5 g

FRUIT AND VEGETABLE BREAD

Caramelized Onion Focaccia Bread

Servings: 4
Cooking Time: 10 Minutes
Ingredients:
- 3/4 cup water
- 2 tablespoons olive oil
- 1 tablespoon sugar
- 1 teaspoon salt
- 2 cups flour
- 1 1/2 teaspoons yeast
- 3/4 cup mozzarella cheese, shredded
- 2 tablespoons parmesan cheese, shredded
- Onion topping:
- 3 tablespoons butter
- 2 medium onions
- 2 cloves garlic, minced

Directions:
1. Preparing the Ingredients
2. Place all ingredients, except cheese and onion topping, in your bread maker in the order listed above. Grease a large baking sheet. Pat dough into a 12-inch circle on the pan; cover and let rise in warm place for about 30 minutes.
3. Melt butter in large frying pan over medium-low heat. Cook onions and garlic in butter 15 minutes, stirring often, until onions are caramelized.
4. Preheat an oven to 400°F.
5. Make deep depressions across the dough at 1-inch intervals with the handle of a wooden spoon. Spread the onion topping over dough and sprinkle with cheeses.
6. Bake 15 to 20 minutes or until golden brown. Cut into wedges and serve warm.

Monkey Bread

Servings: 12 - 15
Cooking Time: 2 Hours
Ingredients:
- 1 cup water
- 1 cup butter, unsalted
- 2 tablespoons butter, softened
- 3 cups all-purpose flour
- 1 teaspoon ground cinnamon

- 1 teaspoon salt
- 1/4 cup white sugar
- 2 1/2 teaspoons active dry yeast
- 1 cup brown sugar, packed
- 1 cup raisins
- Flour, for surface

Directions:
1. Add ingredients, except 1 cup butter, brown sugar, raisins and yeast, to bread maker pan in order listed above.
2. Make a well in the center of the dry ingredients and add the yeast. Make sure that no liquid comes in contact with the yeast.
3. Select Dough cycle and press Start.
4. Place finished dough on floured surface and knead 10 times.
5. Melt one cup of butter in small saucepan.
6. Stir in brown sugar and raisins and mix until smooth. Remove from heat.
7. Cut dough into one inch chunks.
8. Drop one chunk at a time into the butter sugar mixture. Thoroughly coat dough pieces, then layer them loosely in a greased Bundt pan.
9. Let rise in a warm, draft-free space; about 15 to 20 minutes.
10. Bake at 375°F for 20 to 25 minutes or until golden brown.
11. Remove from oven, plate, and serve warm.
Nutrition Info: Calories: 294, Sodium: 265. Mg, Dietary Fiber: 1.3 g, Fat: 14.1 g, Carbs: 40 g, Protein: 3.3 g.

Chocolate-pistachio Bread

Servings: 2/3 Cup (24 Slices)
Cooking Time: 10 Minutes
Ingredients:
- 2/3 cup granulated sugar
- ½ cup butter, melted
- ¾ cup milk
- 1 egg
- 1½ cups all-purpose flour
- 1 cup chopped pistachio nuts
- ½ cup semisweet chocolate chips
- 1/3 cup unsweetened baking cocoa

- 2 teaspoons baking powder
- ¼ teaspoon salt
- Decorator sugar crystals, if desired

Directions:
1. Preparing the Ingredients.
2. Choose the size of loaf of your preference and then measure the ingredients.
3. Add all of the ingredients mentioned previously in the list. Close the lid after placing the pan in the bread machine.
4. Select the Bake cycle
5. Turn on the bread machine. Select the White/Basic setting, select the loaf size, and the crust color. Press start.
6. When the cycle is finished, carefully remove the pan from the bread maker and let it rest.
7. Remove the bread from the pan, put in a wire rack to cool for at least 2 hours. Wrap tightly and store at room temperature up to 4 days, or refrigerate.

Carrot Coriander Bread

Servings: 14 Slices
Cooking Time: 3 H.
Ingredients:
- 2-3 freshly grated carrots,
- 1⅛ cup lukewarm water
- 2 Tbsp sunflower oil
- 4 tsp freshly chopped coriander
- 2½ cups unbleached white bread flour
- 2 tsp ground coriander
- 1 tsp salt
- 5 tsp sugar
- 4 tsp easy blend dried yeast

Directions:
1. Add each ingredient to the bread machine in the order and at the temperature recommended by your bread machine manufacturer.
2. Close the lid, select the basic bread, medium crust setting on your bread machine, and press start.
3. When the bread machine has finished baking, remove the bread and put it on a cooling rack.

Fresh Blueberry Bread

Servings: 1 Loaf

Cooking Time: 10 Minutes
Ingredients:
- 12 to 16 slices (1½ to 2 pounds)
- 1 cup plain Greek yogurt, at room temperature
- ½ cup milk, at room temperature
- 3 tablespoons butter, at room temperature
- 2 eggs, at room temperature
- ½ cup sugar
- ¼ cup light brown sugar
- 1 teaspoon pure vanilla extract
- ½ teaspoon lemon zest
- 2 cups all-purpose flour
- 1 tablespoon baking powder
- ¾ teaspoon salt
- ¼ teaspoon ground nutmeg
- 1 cup blueberries

Directions:
1. Preparing the Ingredients.
2. Place the yogurt, milk, butter, eggs, sugar, brown sugar, vanilla, and zest in your bread machine.
3. Select the Bake cycle.
4. Program the machine for Quick/Rapid bread and press Start. While the wet ingredients are mixing, stir together the flour, baking powder, salt, and nutmeg in a medium bowl. After the first fast mixing is done and the machine signals, add the dry ingredients. When the second mixing cycle is complete, stir in the blueberries. When the loaf is done, remove the bucket from the machine. Let the loaf cool for 5 minutes. Gently shake the bucket to remove the loaf, and turn it out onto a rack to cool.

Cinnamon Raisin Breadsticks

Servings: 16
Cooking Time: 3 Hours
Ingredients:
- 1 cup milk
- 2 tablespoons water
- 1 tablespoon oil
- 3/4 teaspoon salt
- 2 tablespoons brown sugar
- 3 cups bread flour
- 1 teaspoon cinnamon
- 1 tablespoon active dry yeast
- 1/2 cup raisins

- Vanilla icing, for glaze

Directions:
1. Preheat oven to 475°F.
2. Mix the cinnamon into the bread flour.
3. Add milk, water, oil, salt and brown sugar to the bread maker pan, then add the flour/cinnamon mixture.
4. Make a well in the center of the dry ingredients and add the yeast.
5. Set on Dough cycle and press Start.
6. Take out the dough out and punch down; let rest for 10 minutes.
7. Roll dough into a 12-by-8-inch rectangle.
8. Sprinkle raisins on one half of the dough and gently press them into the dough.
9. Fold the dough in half and gently roll and stretch dough back out into a rectangle.
10. Cut into strips, then twist.
11. Line a baking sheet with parchment paper and bake for 4 minutes.
12. Place on 2 baking sheets that have been lined with parchment paper. Reduce oven temperature to 350°F.
13. Brush breadsticks lightly with water and return to oven and bake 20-25 minutes.
14. Cool on a wire rack.
15. Glaze with vanilla icing and serve.

Nutrition Info: Calories: 121, Sodium: 117 mg, Dietary Fiber: 1 g, Fat: 1.4 g, Carbs: 23.7 g, Protein: 3.4 g.

Cocoa Date Bread

Servings: 1 Loaf

Ingredients:
- 16 slice bread (2 pounds)
- 1 cup lukewarm water
- ½ cup lukewarm milk
- 2 tablespoons unsalted butter, melted
- 5 tablespoons honey
- 3 tablespoons molasses
- 1 tablespoon sugar
- 3 tablespoons skim milk powder
- 1 teaspoon table salt
- 2 cups white bread flour
- 2½ cups whole-wheat flour
- 1 tablespoon cocoa powder, unsweetened

- 1½ teaspoons bread machine yeast
- 1 cup dates, chopped
- 12 slice bread (1½ pounds)
- ¾ cup lukewarm water
- ½ cup lukewarm milk
- 2 tablespoons unsalted butter, melted
- ¼ cup honey
- 3 tablespoons molasses
- 1 tablespoon sugar
- 2 tablespoons skim milk powder
- 1 teaspoon table salt
- 1¼ cups white bread flour
- 2¼ cups whole-wheat flour
- 1 tablespoon cocoa powder, unsweetened
- 1½ teaspoons bread machine yeast
- ¾ cup dates, chopped

Directions:
1. Choose the size of loaf you would like to make and measure your ingredients.
2. Add all of the ingredients except for the dates to the bread pan in the order listed above.
3. Place the pan in the bread machine and close the lid.
4. Turn on the bread maker. Select the White/Basic or Fruit/Nut (if your machine has this setting) setting, then the loaf size, and finally the crust color. Start the cycle.
5. When the machine signals to add ingredients, add the dates. (Some machines have a fruit/nut hopper where you can add the dates when you start the machine. The machine will automatically add them to the dough during the baking process.)
6. When the cycle is finished and the bread is baked, carefully remove the pan from the machine. Use a potholder as the handle will be very hot. Let rest for a few minutes.
7. Remove the bread from the pan and allow to cool on a wire rack for at least 10 minutes before slicing.

Nutrition Info: (Per Serving):Calories 221, fat 2.7 g, carbs 38.6 g, sodium 227 mg, protein 4.8 g

Strawberry Shortcake Bread

Servings: 1 Loaf
Cooking Time: 10 Minutes
Ingredients:

- 12 slice bread (1½ pounds)
- 1⅛ cups milk, at 80°F to 90°F
- 3 tablespoons melted butter, cooled
- 3 tablespoons sugar
- 1½ teaspoons salt
- ¾ cup sliced fresh strawberries
- 1 cup quick oats
- 2¼ cups white bread flour
- 1½ teaspoons bread machine or instant yeast

Directions:
1. Preparing the Ingredients.
2. Choose the size of loaf of your preference and then measure the ingredients.
3. Add all of the ingredients mentioned previously in the list. Close the lid after placing the pan in the bread machine.
4. Select the Bake cycle
5. Turn on the bread machine. Select the White/Basic setting, select the loaf size, and the crust color. Press start.
6. When the cycle is finished, carefully remove the pan from the bread maker and let it rest.
7. Remove the bread from the pan, put in a wire rack to cool for at least 2 hours, and slice.

Poppy Seed–lemon Bread

Servings: 1 Loaf
Cooking Time: 10 Minutes
Ingredients:
- 1 cup sugar
- ¼ cup grated lemon peel
- 1 cup milk
- ¾ cup vegetable oil
- 2 tablespoons poppy seed
- 2 teaspoons baking powder
- ½ teaspoon salt
- 2 eggs, slightly beaten

Directions:
1. Preparing the Ingredients.
2. Choose the size of loaf of your preference and then measure the ingredients.
3. Add all of the ingredients mentioned previously in the list. Close the lid after placing the pan in the bread machine
4. Select the Bake cycle

5. Turn on the bread machine. Select the White/Basic setting, select the loaf size, and the crust color. Press start.
6. When the cycle is finished, carefully remove the pan from the bread maker and let it rest.
7. Remove the bread from the pan, put in a wire rack to cool completely, about 2 hours. Wrap tightly and store at room temperature up to 4 days, or refrigerate.

Banana Whole-wheat Bread

Servings: 1 Loaf
Cooking Time: 10 Minutes
Ingredients:
- 12 slice bread (1½ pounds)
- ½ cup milk, at 80°F to 90°F
- 1 cup mashed banana
- 1 egg, at room temperature
- 1½ tablespoons melted butter, cooled
- 3 tablespoons honey
- 1 teaspoon pure vanilla extract
- ½ teaspoon salt
- 1 cup whole-wheat flour
- 1¼ cups white bread flour
- 1½ teaspoons bread machine or instant yeast

Directions:
1. Preparing the Ingredients.
2. Choose the size of loaf of your preference and then measure the ingredients.
3. Add all of the ingredients mentioned previously in the list. Close the lid after placing the pan in the bread machine
4. Select the Bake cycle.
5. Turn on the bread machine. Select the Sweet bread setting, select the loaf size, and the crust color. Press start. When the cycle is finished, carefully remove the pan from the bread maker and let it rest.
6. Shake the bucket to remove the loaf, and turn it out onto a rack to cool.

Cranberry Orange Breakfast Bread

Servings: 14 Slices
Cooking Time: 10 Minutes
Ingredients:
- 1⅛ cup orange juice

- 2 Tbsp vegetable oil
- 2 Tbsp honey
- 3 cups bread flour
- 1 Tbsp dry milk powder
- ½ tsp ground cinnamon
- ½ tsp ground allspice
- 1 tsp salt
- 1 (.25 ounce) package active dry yeast
- 1 Tbsp grated orange zest
- 1 cup sweetened dried cranberries
- ⅓ cup chopped walnuts

Directions:
1. Preparing the Ingredients.
2. Add each ingredient to the bread machine in the order and at the temperature recommended by your bread machine manufacturer.
3. Select the Bake cycle
4. Close the lid, select the basic bread, low crust setting on your bread machine, and press start.
5. Add the cranberries and chopped walnuts 5 to 10 minutes before last kneading cycle ends.
6. When the bread machine has finished baking, remove the bread and put it on a cooling rack.

Harvest Fruit Bread

Servings: 14 Slices
Cooking Time: 3 H.
Ingredients:
- 1 cup plus 2 Tbsp water (70°F to 80°F)
- 1 egg
- 3 Tbsp butter, softened
- ¼ cup packed brown sugar
- 1½ tsp salt
- ¼ tsp ground nutmeg
- Dash allspice
- 3¾ cups plus 1 Tbsp bread flour
- 2 tsp active dry yeast
- 1 cup dried fruit (dried cherries, cranberries and/or raisins)
- ⅓ cup chopped pecans

Directions:
1. Add each ingredient except the fruit and pecans to the bread machine in the order and at the temperature recommended by your bread machine manufacturer.

2. Close the lid, select the basic bread, medium crust setting on your bread machine, and press start.
3. Just before the final kneading, add the fruit and pecans.
4. When the bread machine has finished baking, remove the bread and put it on a cooling rack.

French Onion Bread

Servings: 1 Loaf
Cooking Time: 10 Minutes
Ingredients:
- 12 slice bread (1½ pounds)
- 1¼ cups milk, at 80°F to 90°F
- ¼ cup melted butter, cooled
- 3 tablespoons light brown sugar
- 1 teaspoon salt
- 3 tablespoons dehydrated onion flakes
- 2 tablespoons chopped fresh chives
- 1 teaspoon garlic powder
- 3 cups white bread flour
- 1 teaspoon bread machine or instant yeast

Directions:
1. Preparing the Ingredients.
2. Choose the size of loaf of your preference and then measure the ingredients.
3. Add all of the ingredients mentioned previously in the list.
4. Close the lid after placing the pan in the bread machine.
5. Select the Bake cycle
6. Turn on the bread machine. Select the White/Basic setting, select the loaf size, and the crust color. Press start.
7. When the cycle is finished, carefully remove the pan from the bread maker and let it rest.
8. Remove the bread from the pan, put in a wire rack to Cool about 5 minutes. Slice

Potato Dill Bread

Servings: 14 Slices
Cooking Time: 40 Min.
Ingredients:
- 1 (.25 oz) package active dry yeast
- ½ cup water
- 1 Tbsp sugar

- 1 tsp salt
- 2 Tbsp melted butter
- 1 package or bunch fresh dill
- ¾ cup room temperature mashed potatoes
- 2¼ cups bread flour

Directions:

1. Add each ingredient to the bread machine in the order and at the temperature recommended by your bread machine manufacturer.
2. Close the lid, select the basic bread, medium crust setting on your bread machine, and press start.
3. When the bread machine has finished baking, remove the bread and put it on a cooling rack.

Garden Vegetable Bread

Servings: 14 Slices
Cooking Time: 3 H.

Ingredients:

- ½ cup warm buttermilk (70°F to 80°F)
- 3 Tbsp water (70°F to 80°F)
- 1 Tbsp canola oil
- ⅔ cup shredded zucchini
- ¼ cup chopped red sweet pepper
- 2 Tbsp chopped green onions
- 2 Tbsp grated parmesan cheese
- 2 Tbsp sugar
- 1 tsp salt
- ½ tsp lemon-pepper seasoning
- ½ cup old-fashioned oats
- 2½ cup bread flour
- 1½ tsp active dry yeast
- Peppercorns

Directions:

1. Add each ingredient to the bread machine in the order and at the temperature recommended by your bread machine manufacturer.
2. Close the lid, select the basic bread, medium crust setting on your bread machine and press start.
3. When the bread machine has finished baking, remove the bread and put it on a cooling rack.

Yeasted Carrot Bread

Servings: 1 Loaf
Cooking Time: 10 Minutes

Ingredients:

- 12 slice bread (1½ pounds)
- ¾ cup milk, at 80°F to 90°F
- 3 tablespoons melted butter, cooled
- 1 tablespoon honey
- 1½ cups shredded carrot
- ¾ teaspoon ground nutmeg
- ½ teaspoon salt
- 3 cups white bread flour
- 2¼ teaspoons bread machine or active dry yeast

Directions:

1. Preparing the Ingredients.
2. Choose the size of loaf of your preference and then measure the ingredients.
3. Add all of the ingredients mentioned previously in the list.
4. Close the lid after placing the pan in the bread machine.
5. Select the Bake cycle
6. Turn on the bread machine. Select the Quick/Rapid setting, select the loaf size, and the crust color. Press start.
7. When the cycle is finished, carefully remove the pan from the bread maker and let it rest.
8. Remove the bread from the pan, put in a wire rack to Cool about 5 minutes. Slice

Brown Sugar Date Nut Swirl Bread

Servings: 16
Cooking Time: 2 Hours 30 Minutes

Ingredients:

- 1 cup milk
- 1 large egg
- 4 tablespoons butter
- 4 tablespoons sugar
- 1 teaspoon salt
- 4 cups flour
- 1 2/3 teaspoons yeast
- For the filling:
- 1/2 cup packed brown sugar
- 1 cup walnuts, chopped
- 1 cup medjool dates, pitted and chopped
- 2 teaspoons cinnamon
- 2 teaspoons clove spice
- 1 1/3 tablespoons butter
- Powdered sugar, sifted

Directions:

1. Add wet ingredients to the bread maker pan.
2. Mix flour, sugar and salt and add to pan.
3. Make a well in the center of the dry ingredients and add the yeast.
4. Select the Dough cycle and press Start.
5. Punch the dough down and allow it to rest in a warm place.
6. Mix the brown sugar with walnuts, dates and spices; set aside.
7. Roll the dough into a rectangle, on a lightly floured surface.
8. Baste with a tablespoon of butter, add the filling.
9. Start from the short side and roll the dough to form a jelly roll shape.
10. Place the roll into a greased loaf pan and cover.
11. Let it rise in a warm place, until nearly doubled in size; about 30 minutes.
12. Bake at 350°F for approximately 30 minutes.
13. Cover with foil during the last 10 minutes of cooking.
14. Transfer to a cooling rack for 15 minutes; sprinkle with the powdered sugar and serve.

Nutrition Info: Calories: 227, Sodium: 197 mg, Dietary Fiber: 1.5 g, Fat: 8.3 g, Carbs: 33.1 g, Protein: 5.5 g.

Apple Spice Bread

Servings: 1 Loaf
Cooking Time: 10 Minutes
Ingredients:

- 16 slice bread (2 pounds)
- 1⅓ cup milk, at 80°F to 90°F
- 3⅓ tablespoons melted butter, cooled
- 2⅔ tablespoons sugar
- 2 teaspoons salt
- 1⅓ teaspoons ground cinnamon
- Pinch ground cloves
- 4 cups white bread flour
- 2¼ teaspoons bread machine or active dry yeast
- 1⅓ cups finely diced peeled apple

Directions:

1. Preparing the Ingredients.
2. Choose the size of loaf of your preference and then measure the ingredients.

3. Add all of the ingredients mentioned previously in the list, except for the apple. Close the lid after placing the pan in the bread machine.
4. Select the Bake cycle
5. Turn on the bread machine. White/Basic or Fruit/Nut (if your machine has this setting) setting, select the loaf size, and the crust color. Press start.
6. When the machine signals to add ingredients, add the apple. When the cycle is finished, carefully remove the pan from the bread maker and let it rest.
7. Remove the bread from the pan, put in a wire rack to cool for at least 10 minutes, and slice.

Savory Sweet Potato Pan Bread

Servings: 1 Loaf
Cooking Time: 10 Minutes
Ingredients:

- 8 wedges
- 1½ cups uncooked shredded dark-orange sweet potato (about ½ potato) ½ cup sugar
- ¼ cup vegetable oil
- 2 eggs
- ¾ cup all-purpose flour
- ¾ cup whole wheat flour
- 2 teaspoons dried minced onion
- 1 teaspoon dried rosemary leaves, crumbled
- 1 teaspoon baking soda
- ½ teaspoon salt
- ¼ teaspoon baking powder
- 2 teaspoons sesame seed

Directions:

1. Preparing the Ingredients.
2. Choose the size of loaf of your preference and then measure the ingredients.
3. Add all of the ingredients mentioned previously in the list. Close the lid after placing the pan in the bread machine.
4. Select the Bake cycle
5. Turn on the bread machine. Select the White/Basic setting, select the loaf size, and the crust color. Press start.
6. When the cycle is finished, carefully remove the pan from the bread maker and let it rest.
7. Remove the bread from the pan, put in a wire rack to Cool about 10 minutes. Serve warm.

Yeasted Pumpkin Bread

Servings: 1 Loaf
Cooking Time: 10 Minutes
Ingredients:
- 8 slice bread (1 pounds)
- ⅓ cup milk, at 80°F to 90°F
- ⅔ cup canned pumpkin
- 2 tablespoons melted butter, cooled
- ⅔ teaspoon grated ginger
- 2¾ tablespoons sugar
- ½ teaspoon salt
- ⅔ teaspoon ground cinnamon
- ¼ teaspoon ground cloves
- 2 cups white bread flour
- 1⅛ teaspoons bread machine or instant yeast

Directions:
1. Preparing the Ingredients.
2. Choose the size of loaf of your preference and then measure the ingredients.
3. Add all of the ingredients mentioned previously in the list.
4. Close the lid after placing the pan in the bread machine.
5. Select the Bake cycle
6. Turn on the bread machine. Select the White/Basic setting, select the loaf size, and the crust color. Press start.
7. When the cycle is finished, carefully remove the pan from the bread maker and let it rest.
8. Remove the bread from the pan, put in a wire rack to Cool about 10 minutes. Slice

Cheese Onion Garlic Bread

Servings: 10
Cooking Time: 3 Hours
Ingredients:
- Cheddar cheese – 1 cup., shredded
- Dried onion – 3 tbsps., minced
- Garlic powder – 2 tsps.
- Active dry yeast – 2 tsps.
- Margarine – 2 tbsps.
- Sugar – 2 tbsps.
- Milk Powder – 2 tbsps.
- Bread flour – 3 cups.
- Warm water – 1 1/8 cups.
- Salt – 1 ½ tsps.

Directions:
1. Add water, salt, flour, milk powder, sugar, margarine, and yeast into the bread machine pan. Select basic setting then select medium crust and press start. Add cheese, dried onion, and garlic powder just before the final kneading cycle. Once loaf is done, remove the loaf pan from the machine. Allow it to cool for 10 minutes. Slice and serve.

Appendix : Recipes Index

Printed in the USA
CPSIA information can be obtained
at www.ICGtesting.com
LVHW072005080124
768359LV00008B/889